'An honest and eye-opening exploratic   the lives of people with dementia. I found the key to opening my eyes was the statement that we shouldn't look at the dolls, but look at the person. Enough beneficial examples are given for me to feel comfortable about the judicious use of dolls while empirical investigations tease out who they are good for and under what circumstances.'

– Professor Richard Fleming PhD, Director, NSW/ACT Dementia Training Study Centre, Adjunct Professor, Wicking Dementia Research and Education Centre, University of Tasmania

'For some people the mere mention of doll therapy will induce fears of infantilisation and invalidation, and it will be quickly dismissed as inappropriate. I admire the fact that this author lays out his own initial thoughts of this nature at the start of the book. However, he then goes on to piece together a compelling and well-constructed book that will challenge any practitioner to dismiss this as a valid form of non-pharmacological intervention. The book wrangles with the ethical dilemmas of doll therapy, it uses well-researched evidence and highlights many personal stories. He gives detailed practice examples from some very well-respected services and he ends by offering some very useful practice guidelines. For such an evidence-based book it is an emotionally challenging read and I would encourage anyone in search of the best forms of human intervention for people with dementia and their families to read this. Enjoy the challenge, then make your mind up; I suspect you might change your view by the end.'

– Henry Simmons, Chief Executive, Alzheimer Scotland

'This is a book that is very overdue in the dementia care field… Gary writes in an engaging and accessible style, providing a comprehensive range of theoretical and practical illustrations of why every hospital, care home or day service, where people living with a dementia may find themselves, needs to ensure that dolls are an integral part of their repertoire of approaches. This is a book which has at its core the recognition that the real heart of all our human experiences is the need for love, and when we are facing the many losses and challenges of the journey of dementia, we need to be sure love is there for us even more.'

– Sally Knocker, Consultant Trainer with Dementia Care Matters

'I was asked to review *Doll Therapy in Dementia Care* by Gary Mitchell. To be honest I was reluctant to believe this could be used to alleviate distress or agitation. After reading the book two times as a person who has Alzheimer's and PCA, I thought it was written by a person who clearly had empathy and clearly illustrated how individuals at a later stage of dementia could satisfy their inner feelings of need, being loved and wanted. The most important aspect of care that a family want for their loved ones is ensuring they are content and happy within their environment. It can be very difficult for relatives watching their mum or family member cuddling an inanimate doll. Yet, perceptions can change once they see their "loved one smile with pleasure at holding something close to love again". The image of an older person cuddling and singing to a doll can seem strange and incongruous. Yet I realise I had the same need, and when my grandson was born, I was doing the same thing but instead of being a doll it was a real baby. I couldn't get enough. I had such a yearning to hold, love and want to have this baby as much as I could. The moral and ethical dilemmas should not supersede the reality of the beneficial impact – every person has a vivid desire to express affection, physical nurturing and emotional attachment that is clearly stored in the repository of their brains, irrespective of what type of dementia or stage they are at.'

– Liz Cunningham, person living with dementia and Ambassador and Dementia Friendly Communities Champion for the Alzheimer's Society

'Gary Mitchell has refreshingly delved into controversy, effectively dispelling stereotypical, preconceived judgements surrounding the practice of using dolls in dementia care. Whether regenerating past relationships or regaining the space held in the world, he has provided an impetus to developing an increased open-mindedness in the provision of encounters that encourage positive ageing, this respecting meaningful experiences based on deferential reciprocity. Demonstrating another valuable way forward in the provision of person-centred dementia care and preservation of personhood. Delightful and insightful.'

– Leah Bisiani, Dementia Consultant, MHlthSc, 'Uplifting Dementia', shimmeringspirit.wix.com/uplifting-dementia

DOLL THERAPY IN
DEMENTIA CARE

of related interest

A Creative Toolkit for Communication in Dementia Care
Karrie Marshall
ISBN 978 1 84905 694 6
eISBN 978 1 78450 206 5

Facilitating Spiritual Reminiscence for People with Dementia
A Learning Guide
Elizabeth MacKinlay and Corinne Trevitt
ISBN 978 1 84905 573 4
eISBN 978 1 78450 018 4

Developing Excellent Care for People Living
with Dementia in Care Homes
Caroline Baker
ISBN 978 1 84905 467 6
eISBN 978 1 78450 053 5

Understanding Behaviour in Dementia that Challenges
A Guide to Assessment and Treatment
Ian Andrew James
ISBN 978 1 84905 108 8
eISBN 978 0 85700 296 9

DOLL THERAPY IN DEMENTIA CARE

EVIDENCE AND PRACTICE

GARY MITCHELL

FOREWORD BY SALLY KNOCKER

Jessica Kingsley *Publishers*
London and Philadelphia

First published in 2016
by Jessica Kingsley Publishers
73 Collier Street
London N1 9BE, UK
and
400 Market Street, Suite 400
Philadelphia, PA 19106, USA

www.jkp.com

Library of Congress Cataloging in Publication Data
Names: Mitchell, Gary (Gary George Ernest), 1985- editor.
Title: Doll therapy in dementia care / [edited by] Gary Mitchell.
Description: London ; Philadelphia : Jessica Kingsley Publishers, 2016. |
    Includes bibliographical references and index.
Identifiers: LCCN 2016005892 | ISBN 9781849055703 (alk. paper)
Subjects: LCSH: Dementia--Treatment. | Dolls--Therapeutic use. |
    Dementia--Patients--Rehabilitation.
Classification: LCC RC521 .D65 2016 | DDC 616.89/1653--
dc23 LC record available at http://lccn.loc.gov/2016005892

British Library Cataloguing in Publication Data
A CIP catalogue record for this book is available from the British Library

ISBN 978 1 84905 570 3
eISBN 978 1 78450 007 8

Printed and bound in the United States

Contents

Foreword

I write this foreword on a train journey returning from a care home in Wales where I have spent the afternoon observing the magic of dolls. A woman who had been experiencing some distress as she was asking for her own mother repeatedly was offered a doll to hold. Immediately her face lit up and she started to chat to the baby; 'Aren't you a smasher?' she says. 'You're my best boy!' (She seems refreshingly unperturbed the doll was dressed in pink!) She then proceeds to cuddle and sing to him for the next forty minutes, with no signs of her previous unhappiness. She had found someone to cherish and at once all is well with her world.

There is a danger when we talk about 'therapy'; there is a sense there is something that needs to be fixed. People living with a dementia don't want or need us to 'fix' them; like all of us, they want us to be alongside where they are from moment to moment, to put our own prejudices or assumptions about what might be 'good' or 'not good' for another person aside and to learn and trust the language of emotions.

This is a book that is overdue in the dementia care field. At one level, it surprises me that we still have to justify and evidence an intervention which is so obviously beneficial. Professor Tom Kitwood, whose ground breaking work in dementia care in the 1990s is referred to in this book, described the psychological needs of people living with a dementia as like petals on a flower: the need for attachment, comfort, inclusion or belonging, recognition of identity and the need to be occupied. As the following chapters will describe in detail, a doll can be many things to a person with a dementia: a treasured baby to nurture and protect; a way of communicating a need to others or a projection of their own vulnerable self; a source of companionship, playfulness and comfort; and a way to alleviate loneliness or boredom. Those of us who have walked in a park with a young baby or a dog will know that we are also much more likely to find that people will want to stop and chat with us because there is a focus on our connection, which helps break the ice.

It is no coincidence that at the centre of Tom Kitwood's flower of psychological needs, that around which all the other petals grow is 'love'. With all the current emphasis on smart hotel-style environments and professional standards in many care services, we can sometimes forget the simple truth that when we feel loved and are still able to give love, we are likely not just to survive but to flourish in a care environment.

Gary writes in an engaging and accessible style providing a comprehensive range of theoretical and practical illustrations of why every hospital, care home or day service, where people living with a dementia may find themselves, needs to ensure that dolls are an integral part of their repertoire of approaches. This is a book which has at its core the recognition that the real heart of all our human experiences is the need for love, and when we are facing the many losses and challenges of the journey of dementia, we need to be sure that love is there for us even more.

Sally Knocker
Consultant Trainer with Dementia Care Matters

Acknowledgements

As you will learn, my first experiences of doll therapy in dementia care were quite negative. As a fresh-faced nursing graduate from Queen's University Belfast, I took up my first post within a dementia care unit in early 2010. Over time my feelings on doll therapy began to become more positive, thanks in no small part to my mentor within the dementia care unit at Oakridge Care Home, Sister Elizabeth O'Neill. It was fair to say that Liz was an extremely empathetic practitioner, and without her clinical mentorship I would not have eventually championed doll therapy within dementia care. Throughout my professional career at Four Seasons Health Care, I have also been fortunate to be supported in my understanding of doll therapy and its application to practice, as well as many other aspects of dementia care, by the specialist knowledge of Joanne Agnelli, who was indeed responsible for my first clinical dementia education sessions at the company as well as my continued professional development.

Through my experiences in practice and academia, I have come to appreciate that many people share differing views on a great number of issues. As it pertains to doll therapy in dementia care, opinion is still divided, and this book is my attempt to chronicle the evidence that underpins doll therapy, how it can be applied to a number of advocated theories within the context of person-centred care, bioethics and palliative care, as well as recommending best practice guidelines for operationalising doll therapy in dementia care. In addition, I am honoured to be able to provide reflections on doll therapy from prominent members of the dementia care community.

I reserve special thanks to my co-authors who have taken considerable time to help me shape the contents of this book – thank you Professor Brendan McCormack, Professor Tanya

McCance, Professor Jan Dewing, Professor Ian Andrew James, Ruth Lee and the Newcastle Challenging Behaviour Team, Caroline Baker and Marsha Tuffin. I was especially honoured to have contributions from my own close personal friends Dr Michelle Templeton, Dr Helen Kerr and Jessie McGreevy – again, a special thank you goes out to you. I believe this collective expertise has helped me to provide a balanced and comprehensive overview of doll therapy in dementia care.

I am grateful for the support of Jessica Kingsley Publishers, and in particular my commissioning editor Rachel Menzies. Rachel's enthusiasm and belief in the project greatly assisted in helping me to deliver what is my first attempt at writing a book! I also thank the people behind the scenes at Jessica Kingsley Publishers who have helped make this project a reality.

Finally, I must thank my beautiful (and wonderfully tolerant) wife Claire, our little boy Zachary, my mum Sylvia, dad Trevor and other members of my family and friends. Your combined belief, encouragement and motivation have helped me immensely in the completion of this book.

Introduction

Gary Mitchell

In 2010 I took up my first post in a dementia care unit. My nurse training had already garnished me with a number of experiences in oncology, acute medical admissions, surgery and the emergency room. If I was being honest, my first post in dementia care was only intended to be a stepping-stone until I could take up a post in a hospital. Like many healthcare professionals, I had no specialist dementia care training except what I had learned at university and later within my clinical place of work.

When I began my first post I was fortunate enough to receive extensive person-centred care training, both on the job (through various training courses/mentorship sessions) and off the job (with the use of three books). The books were by Tom Kitwood, Christine Bryden and Dawn Brooker. They all celebrated the meaning of 'living well with dementia'. This shocked me at the time because it seemed quite impossible to me. The ethos of the messages from Kitwood, Bryden and Brooker was person-centred care – treating people living with dementia as unique. Absolutely nothing else would suffice. This was a message I could easily get behind.

Braced with an array of person-centred knowledge, coupled with newly qualified enthusiasm, I began my time in the dementia care unit. As I received a walk-through the unit on my first day, I met Clara and 'Tom'. Clara was an older lady living with dementia. She held tightly to Tom as she walked towards me. The nursing sister of the unit, who was taking me on the walk-through, introduced me to Clara and Tom. I was flabbergasted – Tom was a doll. What happened next made me feel as if I had followed Alice down the rabbit hole – the nursing sister, a dementia specialist nurse with over 15 years' experience, took Tom as though he were a human baby, cradled him, kissed his forehead and diligently gave him back to Clara.

A number of thoughts flew through my head: Was this some sort of test? I could never believe that 'playing with dolls' would do much to expel the stigma of people treating those with dementia like children – the precise message of ALL of my dementia training. Had the nursing sister missed the whole point of person-centred care? Doll therapy was infantile, it was patronising. It was just embarrassing. I left the unit that evening with my head exploding…and I confess, when I returned home from the unit, I told my friends and family about the incident with the doll, and we all reached the same conclusion – that I should protect my nursing registration first and foremost, disassociate myself from the practice of 'doll therapy', and begin to look for another clinical position.

Surprisingly, six months passed by, and I still held the position of a dementia care nurse on the unit. The six months had been one hell of a steep learning curve. When I was left in charge of the dementia care unit, I initially removed Tom. But when the nursing sister worked on the opposite shift, Tom returned. This carried on back and forth, until a warm day in July 2010. I was accompanying Clara to the dining room to serve her dinner when suddenly she screamed. Tom was propped up against a window in a vacated resident's room. The door had been left ajar and this had allowed Clara to spot Tom. I remember that she was hysterically calling, 'Tom is going to fall.' Opting for reality orientation (assisting Clara to be aware of her current surroundings; see Chapter 1), I told Clara, as I did many, many times, that Tom was just a doll for children. Like the many, many times before, this served to distress Clara even more because this simply wasn't her reality. I resisted reuniting the pair for a time that day, which incidentally resulted in Clara refusing to eat her lunch, crying quite uncontrollably throughout the day, and generally being in a state of increased illbeing. I simply couldn't justify that I was providing good dementia care anymore. My principles of person-centredness were offset by the distress Clara was experiencing. I began, six months later, to sense that I was missing the point of person-centred dementia care.

Clara's reaction was so distressing that I was forced to reunite the pair later that day. When I did, everything changed in that moment; Clara's smile was instantly back, she enjoyed her evening meal, and engaged with many of the other residents in the unit. This enhanced wellbeing was so visible, so authentic and so real. As I left the shift that night Clara motioned as if to call me over... quite truthfully I thought I was going to be scolded for denying her interaction with Tom earlier in the day.

'How are you doing Clara?' I asked, and she responded in a soft voice, 'Shhhh...baby is sleeping.' I stared at Clara for a second or two. I was going to recite my usual message, 'That is not a real baby, that is a doll for children.' But on that day, for the first time since I began my post, I did not. While I was reflecting on doll therapy I stood in silence looking at Clara when she said to me, 'It is not me you should be looking at, it is him.'

As I was driving away from the unit that night I thought about Clara's words and concluded that she had it wrong – I had indeed been looking at Tom, the doll, all along. It was the doll that represented something that I could not warm to and that I resisted even trying to understand. Then, I was hit by a eureka moment. It was like a person-centred epiphany, if there is such a thing; all this time I had been looking at the doll when I should have been looking at the person...all that time I was looking at Tom, when I should have been looking at Clara.

Throughout my clinical practice I have always tried to do what is best for patients, residents, any person living with an illness, their family and care partners, and my experiences with doll therapy have been my hardest lesson in healthcare to date. For six months I denied Clara something that brought her great joy because I, a registered nurse, did not feel that it was morally right or appropriate. And I was not the only person who was against doll therapy; a number of my colleagues agreed, as well as numerous visitors to the unit. Clara's family were unable to visit the unit often, but they did not have much of a problem with doll therapy. They believed that if engaging with a doll brought Clara happiness, then it was okay with them...it is true that the person living with dementia and their family are almost always the experts.

Through my personal experiences using doll therapy in dementia care, I know that there is limited awareness and understanding about what doll therapy actually is and how it can be used effectively for people living with dementia. Today it is considered a 'controversial' therapy, and is often absent from the literature or practice guidelines when considering other effective therapies or non-pharmacological interventions that can be used within dementia care. It is often started or withheld based on the assumptions or education of the clinician in charge. In relation to non-healthcare settings, and based on my personal experience, there are not many non-clinicians who know that 'doll therapy' actually exists. Unfortunately there is limited reference to doll therapy in dementia care in the literature from charities, policies or practice guidelines worldwide.

To understand more about doll therapy in dementia care, you have to trawl the internet for published blogs, newspaper articles or journal accounts of how it can be effective. My personal and profound experiences in using doll therapy in dementia care have inspired me to write this, my first book with Jessica Kingsley Publishers. The aim of this book, the first of its kind, is to provide an overview of doll therapy in dementia care for all grades and specialities of healthcare workers, as well as for the families and care partners of those living with dementia.

In short, doll therapy is when a person living with dementia engages with a doll, and this engagement comes in a variety of forms. In Clara's case this was holding the doll, talking to the doll, cuddling or hugging the doll, feeding the doll and dressing the doll. The benefits Clara associated with doll therapy include increased levels of engagement with other people, reduction in episodes of distress, improved dietary intake and generally an increased level of wellbeing. And the therapeutic use of doll therapy has been growing globally, with accounts of its use in the UK, Australia, Japan and the USA.

Of course not everyone living with dementia will engage or even benefit from doll therapy, but there is no way to know if a person will derive benefit or not until it is facilitated. It appears, however, that people living in the advanced stages of dementia are the biggest users of doll therapy. The reason for this may be related to the need for attachment in a time of greater uncertainty. For those living with dementia, a doll can arguably act as an anchor in an ever-changing sea of uncertainty.

This book has been written so that each chapter can be read as a stand-alone piece. Naturally, however, reading the book in its entirety is recommended so that all the elements and themes of doll therapy in dementia care can fuse together.

The following is a synopsis of the chapters of this book:

- Chapter 1 provides a general introduction to dementia, the manifestations of the dementia diseases, and the move away from pharmacological interventions and how doll therapy itself is framed within the context of a non-pharmacological intervention that should be promoted and explored within dementia care.

- Chapter 2 provides a thematic overview of the research that is currently available in relation to doll therapy within dementia care. This evidence details how and where doll therapy can be practised, who can facilitate and participate in it, what the benefits and barriers of doll therapy usually are, and why it can work from a theoretical point of view.

- Chapter 3 presents Tom Kitwood's work, and considers how doll therapy, if practised correctly, can be a person-centred approach to dementia care. It also highlights how poor practice of doll therapy can actually perpetuate the stigma associated with the dementia diseases.

- Chapter 4 looks at the ongoing ethical debate that has always been associated with doll therapy. It considers the argument from those who are in favour of doll therapy and those who are not, before providing care partners and healthcare providers with practical assistance in negotiating the potential dilemmas.

- Chapter 5 provides a background on the importance of palliative care in dementia and explores, probably for the first time, how doll therapy can be considered a therapeutic tool within this ethos.

- Chapter 6 illustrates the important role of the Newcastle Doll Therapy Programme, which has greatly informed and shaped practice as it pertains to using doll therapy in dementia care. Indeed, the Newcastle team are considered the global experts in relation to the research they have published on doll therapy in dementia care.

- Chapter 7 is a thoughtful account of a family member's experience of their loved one using doll therapy within a dementia care facility. It highlights how personal feelings of doll therapy can evolve over time.

- Chapters 8 and 9 provide reflections from senior dementia care leaders within the care sector.

- Chapter 10 concludes this book, offering recommendations for healthcare providers, family members and care partners for implementing doll therapy within their practice.

I truly hope that you find this book both useful and enjoyable. Naturally, I dedicate it to all those who live with dementia, their family, friends and care partners. It is my sincere hope that it will help some of those people living with dementia to live better through engagement with doll therapy.

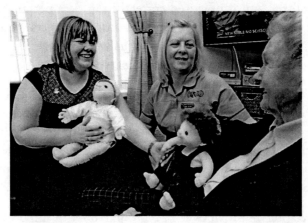

Joanne Agnelli, dementia specialist for Four Seasons Health Care, engages in doll therapy with a resident and a care assistant from Castle Lodge Care Home in Northern Ireland

Chapter 1

Dementia and Society

Gary Mitchell

This chapter provides an overview of dementia within society today. It highlights the prevalence of dementia, the main types of dementia, and the symptoms that are associated with the dementia diseases. It goes on to provide important contextual information about pharmacological and non-pharmacological approaches to dementia care that provide a platform for the discussion of doll therapy in subsequent chapters.

Background

It is estimated that approximately 44 million people in the world are living with dementia (ADI 2014). As global life expectancy continues to increase, and dementia is a disease that is most common in people over 65, it is also estimated that by 2030 these numbers are set to double and by 2050 more than triple. This alarming prediction is compounded by the reality that there is currently no known cure for dementia.

Dementia is a medical term used to describe a number of cognitive syndromes that include Alzheimer's disease, vascular dementia, dementia with Lewy bodies and frontotemporal dementia. These dementia syndromes have common symptoms that occur as the disease progresses, and can include short-term memory loss, impairment of normal social functioning, language deterioration, difficulty in performing automated tasks, communication difficulties, problems with spatial awareness and changes in personality (Ballard *et al.* 2011). The symptoms are variable depending on the type of dementia and the stage of disease. It is important to acknowledge that they are caused by brain disease, and dementia is not part of normal ageing.

While there is continued research on finding a pharmacological cure for the different types of dementia, there is now, perhaps more than ever, an emphasis on finding ways to improve social functioning, enhance levels of wellbeing and reduce episodes of distress within the dementia care arena.

Types of dementia

There are over 100 types of dementia, but most are relatively uncommon. The four main types of dementia – Alzheimer's disease (50–75%), vascular dementia (20–30%), dementia with Lewy bodies (5–20%) and frontotemporal dementia (5–10%) – account for about 90–95 per cent of all dementia cases (Draper 2013). Other neurodegenerative diseases that are classed as dementia but are less common include Parkinson's disease and Huntington's disease. The four main types of dementia are now considered.

Alzheimer's disease

Alzheimer's disease is the most common of all dementias. It is named after German neurologist Alois Alzheimer who first discovered the disease over 100 years ago. Alzheimer's disease occurs as a result of abnormalities that occur in the structure of the brain. These changes cause a change in the physical structure of the brain and its brain chemistry. Alzheimer's disease is progressive, with an average life expectancy of ten years, although this is variable depending on the person.

Vascular dementia

Vascular dementia differs from the other main types of dementia in that it does not follow a predictive course that leads to the progressive death of nerve cells over time. It occurs when blood vessels in the brain become damaged and optimum levels of blood oxygen no longer reach all parts of the brain. The symptoms of vascular dementia can occur quite suddenly, for example, after a stroke, or over a longer period of time, for example, after a number of transient ischaemic attacks (TIAs, or mini-strokes). The damage to these vessels can occur in any part of the brain and so symptoms will depend on the part of the brain that is damaged. Unlike Alzheimer's disease, people living with vascular dementia may see their symptoms stabilise between occurrences of cerebral vascular episodes and not appear to deteriorate in the same manner. After a cerebral vascular episode, the person living with vascular dementia is likely to see a sudden decline in his level of functioning.

Dementia with Lewy bodies

Dementia with Lewy bodies can occur quite suddenly in comparison with Alzheimer's disease. The Lewy bodies are small abnormal structures that develop inside the nerve cells and this causes the destruction of healthy brain tissue. This form of dementia is associated with Parkinson's disease as specific symptoms include tremors, muscle rigidity and a stooped gait. In addition, people living with dementia with Lewy bodies often experience hallucinations as well as difficulties with planning and problem solving, although their memory may be affected to a lesser degree.

Frontotemporal dementia

Frontotemporal dementia includes Pick's disease, and as the name suggests, it is usually focused on damage in the front part of the brain. The frontal lobe is the area responsible for social behaviour, insight, personality and judgement, and personality and behaviour changes are initially the most obvious signs of such a dementia. Pick's disease is caused by abnormal amounts or types of a nerve cell protein, Pick bodies, which cause the degeneration of nerve cells, resulting in shrinkage of the brain tissue.

It is possible for two or more dementias to occur at the same time, for example Alzheimer's disease and vascular disease can occur in up to 25 per cent of cases, and Alzheimer's disease and dementia with Lewy bodies can occur in up to 15 per cent of cases due to the differing ways that these dementia diseases impact on the brain.

Clinical manifestations of dementia

There are numerous clinical manifestations, or symptoms, that are associated with dementia. The specific clinical manifestations depend on the type of dementia, the part of the brain affected and the stage of the disease, so providing a comprehensive list of symptoms can be difficult (Rahman 2014). As dementia is a progressive disease it is helpful to broadly outline what kinds of symptoms manifest over the course of early, middle and later stages of dementia.

Early stages of dementia:

- short-term memory loss

- difficulty in finding the right words

- subtle personality and behavioural changes

- short periods (lasting from minutes to hours) of confusion, disorientation and distress.

Middle stages of dementia:

- severe memory dysfunction

- disorientation to time and place

- difficulty in comprehension

- disinhibition

- major reduction in capacity

- deterioration in ability to self-care

- difficulties in taking long periods of sleep

- increasing periods of distress.

Later stages of dementia:

- requirement for 24-hour care

- inability to recall even most recent events

- inaccurate recollection of past memories

- higher levels of distraction

- rapid loss of language skills

- rapid loss of any ability to self-care

- increased periods of inactivity and despondence

- major decreases in appetite and eating

- high levels of distress.

Pharmacological treatments for dementia

While there are no known cures for the most common types of dementia discussed in this chapter, there are recommended pharmacological treatments that are available that can help decelerate its progression. According to the National Institute for Health and Care Excellence (NICE 2011), the pharmacological treatments recommended for Alzheimer's disease are two-fold: cholinesterase inhibitors and antiglutamergic therapy.

Cholinesterase inhibitors, such as Donepezil, Galantamine and Rivastigmine, are recommended for use in the early to middle stages of dementia. These classes of medication work by slowing the breakdown of certain chemicals (acetylcholine) in the nerves, thereby reducing the abnormal brain chemistry that causes changes to the brain structure. While there have been empirical reports of benefits of cholinesterase inhibitor use in vascular dementia and dementia with Lewy bodies, evidence is not strong enough for them to be recommended outside of Alzheimer's disease. On average, about one in three people living with Alzheimer's disease will have a temporary improvement in their cognition for between one year and 18 months, one in three will stabilise for about the same period, and the remaining one in three will derive no benefit from this class of medications (Draper 2013). There is no significant difference in the effectiveness of the three medications (Mitchell 2013).

There is currently only one medication that has been approved for antiglutamergic therapy, and this is Memantine. The most notable therapeutic effects of Memantine are usually noted in the later stages of dementia. It is therefore recommended for people living with Alzheimer's disease in the middle to late stage (NICE 2011). Memantine works by providing protection from glutamate, a chemical that is released in excessive amounts during Alzheimer's disease that alters normal brain chemistry (Mitchell 2013).

Distress

The manifestation of distress, sometimes termed 'challenging behaviour', 'disruptive behaviour' or 'behaviour that challenges', is unfortunately a common experience for people living with dementia. Distress can occur at any stage of the dementia disease, and can be a difficult obstacle to overcome for people with dementia, their care partners, family and healthcare givers. Like the terms 'challenging behaviour' or 'behaviour that challenges', distress can denote a broad range of things that may include anxiety, anger, depression, fear or suspicion, excessive walking (sometimes termed 'wandering', but this is not the term that we should use), uncooperative behaviour in relation to receiving personal assistance or repeated shouting, to name but a few. Distress can be a consequence of any number of things, but it is usually as a result of interactions between the person living with dementia and another person. It is estimated that this occurs in around 60–90 per cent of people with dementia (James *et al.* 2008).

The term 'distress' is preferable to terms such as 'challenging behaviour' as this can be quite labelling and enhance the stigma already associated with the dementia diseases (Baker 2014). Another slightly more preferable term is that of 'behavioural and psychological symptoms of dementia' (BPSD). While the use of differing terminology might appear pedantic, it is important to reinforce because the language that we, as a society, use can enhance the stigma associated with dementia, and serve to disempower people living with it (Swaffer 2014).

Notable examples of other terms that should not be used include:

- referring to people living with dementia as 'sufferers' or 'victims'

- referring to people living with dementia as 'demented'

- referring to people living with dementia as 'elderly mentally infirm'

- referring to older people as 'elderly'

- referring to walking as 'wandering'.

Pharmacological approaches to distress

With a high prevalence of distress noted among many people living with dementia, it is understandable that there has been a range of empirical investigation and research around what works best in reducing episodes that cause distress. Understandably the reduction of distressing episodes will likely enhance the wellbeing and relationships of those living with dementia, their family, care partners or healthcare providers. We will now explore some pharmacologicial approaches to alleviating distress and enhancing wellbeing in dementia care, including medications for pain, depression, anxiety and distress.

Analgesia

Many people living with dementia are either not recognised as having pain or not receiving effective treatment, and it is estimated that 50 per cent of older adults living with dementia in nursing home settings have been identified as having pain, but approximately only half receive pharmacological treatment for pain relief (Jones and Mitchell 2015). Evidence suggests that healthcare professionals do not often recognise when a person living with dementia is experiencing pain because of the difficulties those with dementia sometimes experience when communicating. This pain can sometimes then manifest as distress (Cohen-Mansfield 2008). The use of a validated pain assessment (such as the Abbey Pain Scale[1]) and regular administration of analgesia are likely to safeguard against pain or reduce its impact for people living with dementia. The form of pain relief will depend on the type of pain, but often in the later stages of dementia, where the person may have difficulty in swallowing his tablets, an analgesic patch (such as Buprenorphine) can be applied every 72 hours, with very good effect. The importance of analgesia should not be underestimated because pain is often the key reason why people living with dementia exhibit distress. When a person living with dementia exhibits distress, always consider the likelihood of pain, determine the likelihood of pain in that person, administer analgesia if appropriate, and monitor the wellbeing of that person to see if the distress diminishes.

Antidepressant medication

The use of antidepressant medication (such as Sertraline, Citalopram, Mirtazapine and Fluoxetine) is used mostly for depression and anxiety. While depression is often a risk factor for all people experiencing a progressive illness, the use of antidepressant medication in dementia is not always effective (Banerjee *et al.* 2013). This is because the brain damage already caused by dementia can often reduce the therapeutic effectiveness of the medication. While antidepressant medication can make a positive difference to some people living with dementia, there may be a risk of side-effects that include nausea, vomiting, diarrhoea, increased risk of falls and sodium imbalance (which can lead to confusion). So the use of antidepressant medication should be used with caution and regularly reviewed with input from the person living with dementia, his care partner and/or a validated assessment tool (such as the Cornell Scale for Depression in Dementia[2]).

---

1   See http://prc.coh.org/PainNOA/Abbey_Tool.pdf

2   See http://geropsychiatriceducation.vch.ca/docs/edu-downloads/depression/cornell_scale_depression.pdf

Anxiolytic and hypnotic medication

The use of anxiolytic medication (such as Diazepam and Lorazepam) and hypnotic medication (such as Temazepam and Zopiclone) are frequently prescribed to alleviate against potential episodes of distress in dementia. Anxiolytic medications are used to reduce anxiety, which can lead to episodes of distress in dementia care, while hypnotic medications are mainly used for sleep disturbances. While these medications can be beneficial in reducing distress in dementia care, they should be used with caution as there a strong chance that they will cause over-sedation. It is important to note that these medications are usually only recommended for short-term use, as long-term use is associated with intolerance and as such, reduced therapeutic effect.

Antipsychotic medication

Antipsychotic medications (such as Risperidone, Quetiapine, Olanzapine and Haloperidol) were originally designed for use in some types of mental health conditions like schizophrenia or bipolar disorder. The psychotic symptoms that these antipsychotic medications target are feelings of suspiciousness, delusions, paranoia and hallucinations. While dementia is not considered in the same bracket as schizophrenia or bipolar disorder (due to its progressive clinical features that are evident in brain tissue), antipsychotic medications are frequently prescribed to people living with dementia who experience significant distress (Sturdy *et al.* 2012).

Antipsychotic medications are extremely beneficial to some people living with dementia, although the evidence suggests that currently these medications are significantly over-prescribed. A report for the Department of Health in the UK estimated that 180,000 people in the UK are prescribed antipsychotic medications, but that approximately only 36,000 of these will derive any therapeutic benefit (Banerjee 2009). This means, on average, that only 20 per cent of people living with dementia (or one in five) who are prescribed antipsychotic medications actually benefit from this form of medication. Sustained administration of antipsychotic medications can be associated with adverse effects, which include accelerated cognitive decline, increased risk of fall, over-sedation, Parkinsonian symptoms and increased risk of developing cardiac problems (James *et al.* 2008). Despite these risk factors, coupled with issues around over-prescription, it is somewhat surprising that Risperidone is actually the only licenced antipsychotic medication for use in people living with dementia for the sole reason of distress, and it is only recommended for a period of up to six weeks (Banerjee 2009). In short, antipsychotic medication should be an absolutely last resort for people living with dementia.

Non-pharmacological approaches to dementia care[3]

Due to the clinical manifestations of the dementia diseases, it is probable that the person experiencing the disease may have some feelings of anxiety, depression, despondency, lethargy and distress, and pharmacological intervention may be necessary to alleviate these symptoms. However, with the exception of analgesia, it is usually recommended that healthcare providers and care partners try non-pharmacological approaches first, as these can often be enough to reduce episodes of distress and also lead to sustained levels of wellbeing. Prescription of analgesia is the exception to this, and should be considered as a first-line treatment when pain is suspected as being a possible cause of distress. The following are some types of non-pharmacological approaches that are popular within dementia care.

Cognitive stimulation therapy

Cognitive stimulation therapy is an intervention that can benefit people, particularly those in the early to moderate stages, living with dementia. It is a recurring group activity with a range of activities that serve to provide a source of cognitive stimulation for people living with dementia. These activities generally focus on concentration or memory, as its purpose is to enhance cognitive and social functioning. Of the non-pharmacological approaches on offer, this is the only one currently recommended by NICE (2006).

3   This section is adapted from Mitchell and Agnelli (2015a).

According to a recent Cochrane review of clinical trials, it has the potential to decelerate dementia disease progression as much as the prescription of cholinesterase inhibitors, such as Donepezil, Galantamine and Rivastigmine (Woods *et al.* 2012).

Reminiscence therapy

Reminiscence therapy focuses on assisting the person living with dementia to relive positive past experiences of his life, for example, his family life, his wedding day, and the places he used to visit or the activities he used to carry out at work. Reminiscence can occur through directed communication or through engagement with stimuli, for example, looking at photographs, reading old books or newspapers or listening to music that holds memories for the person. For it to be effective there is an onus on family, care partners and healthcare providers to find out personal, meaningful details about the person in order to facilitate reminiscence.

Reality orientation

Reality orientation is one of the most widely used non-pharmacological approaches adopted by healthcare providers when attempting to alleviate distress experienced by people living with dementia. Its main aim is to re-orientate the person living with dementia to his current environment (Moniz-Cook 2006). Due to the clinical manifestations of the disease, people living with dementia may become unaware of their surroundings, particularly in long-term care settings that they do not recognise. Reality orientation is a means to alleviate potential distress, and is achieved by orientating the person living with dementia to his current place, date and time. It can be achieved directly through communication between healthcare providers and people living with dementia. Arguably, more subtle reality orientation approaches are also as effective, for example, with adaptions to a care environment, such as prominent displays of clocks or calendars throughout a unit. The use of specialist dementia care signage, such as FIND[4] or

---

4   See http://findsignage.co.uk

Caring Signs[5] (which is popular in the UK), is also recommended as it directs people living with dementia on the unit to nearby lounges, bathrooms or dining rooms (Mitchell and Agnelli 2015a). The personalisation of the person's bedroom, through meaningful photographs, recognisable objects and memory boxes, have also proven effective strategies in relation to reality orientation (Baker 2014).

It should be acknowledged that there are some potential challenges in relation to reality orientation, namely, that the person living with dementia may be experiencing a different reality than the one that is being presented in their care setting. For example, if a displayed calendar states that the year is 2015 and the person living with dementia believes it is 1965, this may cause the person to become distressed. Another example might be if the person resides in a care home and he believes himself to still be at home. When reality orientation techniques appear to cause distress, care partners and healthcare providers should try validation therapy.

Validation therapy

Validation therapy was developed by Naomi Feil (1982) and has been a popular approach in dementia care. It centres on the idea of acceptance of another's reality, and is about providing a high level of empathy as care partners and healthcare professionals to understand a person's entire frame of reference. When considering this therapy, Feil (1982, 1993) postulated that it was an approach that had the potential to alleviate distress as it helped others to understand the reasons that caused distress from the perspective of the person living with dementia. When a care partner or healthcare professional fails to validate a person's feelings or reality, this can intensify the level of distress the person is experiencing.

Music therapy

Music therapy is categorised as a sensory therapy (Bidewell and Chang 2014). It can be receptive (e.g. listening to music) or participatory (e.g. playing a musical instrument or singing along

---

5   See www.caringsigns.co.uk

to songs; see Gold 2014). It is important to personalise music therapy to avoid or manage any distressed reactions. This has been made much easier today with advances in technology, so that dementia care units are able to provide personalised CDs or music playlists on portable media players for a relatively low cost. It is a popular approach to alleviate distress and enhance the wellbeing of people living with dementia because of its ease of use. Music therapy can occur in a communal space, such as a lounge in order to promote relaxation, or it can occur in a dining room, where it has been shown to improve nutritional intake, or even during a bath, to make the experience more therapeutic.

Horticultural therapy

Horticultural, or garden, therapy is a non-pharmacological approach to care that has been flourishing in recent years. It can be directed by care partners or healthcare professionals in a garden area, and activities may be guided, for example, potting up plants, sowing seeds or feeding birds (Blake and Mitchell 2016). It should also be noted that for horticultural therapy to work, care partners or healthcare professionals do not necessarily need to be involved – simply enabling a person to take some of his time in an open garden space can be therapeutic on its own. On a practical note, care partners or healthcare providers have key duties in relation to facilitating horticultural therapy, which pertain to providing routine access to a garden or an outdoors area that has been appropriately risk assessed. Horticultural therapy is social as it enables people living with dementia to engage with others through shared communication (e.g. discourse about the weather), shared activity (e.g. potting up plants), or shared leisure (e.g. eating and drinking together in a garden area).

Pet therapy

Building on the evidence base for attachment and the importance of relationships in dementia care, pet therapy, sometimes known as animal assisted therapy, has shown some positive results. Facilitating interactions, engagement or visits from animals can reduce episodes of distress, use of antipsychotic medication, increase cognitive function and reduce anxiety. While there is no evidence to suggest one type of animal is better than another, dogs tend to be the most widely used in long-term care settings. Although it can be difficult to organise pet therapy in long-term care settings due to issues around infection control, given the potential for therapeutic gain, it is an approach to care that can positively impact those living with dementia (Baker 2014). When considering infection control issues, pet therapy usually only occurs for a short period (e.g. 1–2 hours every week), and is facilitated by someone who is suitably trained (so as to maintain the safety of the people living with dementia). Pet therapy may not be appropriate for everyone, however, particularly if a person living with dementia has a fear or has had negative experiences with animals previously.

Doll therapy

Doll therapy is a non-pharmacological approach in the maintenance of wellbeing or alleviation of distress for some people living with dementia. Doll therapy is when a person living with dementia engages with a doll, and this engagement comes in a variety of forms that might include holding the doll, talking to the doll, cuddling or hugging the doll, feeding the doll or dressing the doll (Mitchell 2014a). This engagement has been associated with a number of benefits for some people with dementia that include increased levels of engagement with others, reduction in episodes of distress and an increased level of wellbeing. In light of the potential benefits associated with doll therapy, its use in clinical practice has been growing globally.

Conclusion

This chapter has provided a brief background to dementia care. The most prevalent types of dementia have been highlighted (Alzheimer's disease, vascular dementia, dementia with Lewy bodies and frontotemporal dementia) along with the clinical manifestations (or symptoms) of dementia throughout the trajectory of the disease (categorised as early, middle and late stages). One of the most common symptoms throughout all stages of dementia is distress, and this was considered along with appropriate pharmacological interventions (including Donepezil, Galantamine, Rivastigmine and Memantine) and less appropriate pharmacological interventions (in some cases medications for depression, anxiety, night sedation and psychosis). The chapter concluded by looking at some of the more widely used non-pharmacological interventions in dementia.

Chapter 2

A Review of the Empirical Evidence[1]

Gary Mitchell, Brendan McCormack and Tanya McCance

This chapter provides an updated version of a systematic literature review on the use of doll therapy in dementia care that was originally carried out by the authors (see Mitchell *et al.* 2014). The 14 empirical studies included in this chapter have been quality assessed by the authors, using the CASP (Critical Appraisal Skills Programme) tool, in order to present healthcare providers with an overview of the current evidence that exists in relation to using doll therapy in dementia care. A range of anecdotal accounts by the likes of Moore (2001), Verity (2006) and Heathcote and Clare (2014), who have written about the personal experiences of doll therapy for people living with dementia, but who have not carried out empirical investigation, are not included in this review.

Activities of daily living

The activities of daily living model has been used by healthcare providers, namely nurses, for a number of years (Roper, Logan and Tierney 2000). Activities of daily living refer to a person's ability to carry out a range of functions and include maintaining a safe environment, communicating, breathing, eating and drinking, elimination (being able to use the toilet), washing and dressing, controlling temperature, mobilisation, working and playing, expressing sexuality, sleeping and dying. These activities are

1 This chapter is adapted and updated from Mitchell, McCormack and McCance (2014).

usually assessed by healthcare providers on admission to a hospital ward or care home, and are reviewed as necessary. This is worth highlighting because people living with dementia gradually experience a decline in these abilities over time. The findings in this chapter are framed with these activities of daily living in mind because, as this chapter will demonstrate, doll therapy has the potential to improve levels of independence in relation to these activities of daily living.

Benefits of doll therapy

All studies included in this review clearly articulated a number of benefits associated with doll therapy. The most common reported benefit was improvement in communication between the person living with dementia and other residents or care staff (Alander, Prescott and James 2013; Bisiani and Angus 2013; Ellingford, Mackenzie and Marsland 2007; Fraser and James 2008; James *et al.* 2006; Mackenzie *et al.* 2006; Minshull 2009; Stephens, Cheston and Gleeson 2013; Tamura, Nakajima and Nambu 2001). The use of dolls gave people living with dementia a means to engage with care staff or residents. In the study by James *et al.* (2006), it was reported that a group of women who engaged with their dolls began to sit together and connect as a group. James *et al.* (2006, p.1095) reported that this group began what was affectionately known as the 'mother's group'. In addition, Minshull (2009) reported that some of her participants actually began to better articulate their language and as a result express themselves more clearly to others. In one example, Minshull (2009, p.37) recalls how one particular person living with dementia was 'normally incoherent in speech' pre-doll therapy. Post-doll therapy, Minshull (2009, p.37) reported that this same person was able to better articulate her language through the doll by communicating phrases like 'baby...tickle her toes...oh pretty colours [regarding doll's pink cardigan]'. The re-establishment of these communication channels is arguably essential when considering the therapeutic relationship between the person living with dementia and healthcare professionals. This notion was supported in Fraser and James' findings (2008), who conducted semi-structured interviews with health professionals that included representation from nursing, psychology, occupational therapy and psychiatry. Fraser and James (2008) identified communication as an important theme as healthcare professionals were able to establish new communication channels with people in their care. They proposed that healthcare professionals were able to use the doll as a starting point for communication, and even talk to the doll and the person living with dementia as means of further developing the therapeutic relationship.

While improvements in communication were important, other activities of daily living were shown to be enhanced through engagement with dolls (Roper *et al.* 2000). Considering maintenance of a safe environment, many studies reported reductions in distressing behaviour experienced by people living with dementia (Bisiani and Angus 2013; Braden and Gaspar 2014; Fraser and James 2008; James *et al.* 2006; Mackenzie *et al.* 2006; Shin 2015; Stephens *et al.* 2013). This distressing behaviour has been mainly described in the literature as agitation, wandering, anxiety, despondency and disengagement from others. During a single case study on the phenomenon, Bisiani and Angus (2013, p.456) illustrated how one resident's (Mary) previous daily experiences of 'trying to leave the facility and asking for attachment/child were all together eradicated' by doll therapy. This was supported by Green *et al.*'s work (2011), who noted that the prescription of certain antipsychotic medications was reduced in those who engaged with dolls.

An improvement in dietary intake, or the activity of eating and drinking, was also identified as a potential benefit of doll therapy (Bisiani and Angus 2013; Braden and Gaspar 2014; Mackenzie *et al.* 2006; Stephens *et al.* 2013). This increased dietary intake was as a result of a better dining experience (as the doll provided immediate company) and increased awareness about food (as the person would sometimes give her own doll food). The studies in this review also found that residents who were previously reluctant to be assisted with elimination and washing/dressing needs were more approachable when engaging with a doll (Bisiani and Angus 2013; Fraser and James 2008; James *et al.* 2006; Mackenzie *et al.* 2006; Stephens *et al.* 2013). The rationale behind this was related to the calming affect that the doll appeared to have on users. Indeed, through analysis of questionnaires administered to healthcare professionals, Mackenzie *et al.* (2006, p.443) found that the most common change in 'emotional status' observed in people engaging with doll therapy was that of being 'calmer'.

Finally, benefits associated with working and playing, sleeping and mobilisation were also described in the literature. According to the findings of this review, therapeutic engagement with dolls has given rise to a number of behaviours including touch, cradling, cuddling, kissing, carrying, talking and singing (Alander *et al.* 2013; Bisiani and Angus 2013; Cohen-Mansfield 2010; Ellingford *et al.* 2007; Fraser and James 2008; James *et al.* 2006; Mackenzie *et al.* 2006; Minshull 2009; Stephens *et al.* 2013; Tamura *et al.* 2001). These behaviours are perceived as therapeutic and not unlike those that would be associated with play therapy. However, as illustrated by Bisiani and Angus (2013), some people who engage with doll therapy are also meeting working needs. For example, Mary was observed to be asking healthcare professionals to 'babysit' when she had other tasks that needed to be carried out (p.456). Improvement in the quality of sleep was another benefit identified by two studies in the literature (Bisiani and Angus 2013; Stephens *et al.* 2013). Presumably, a person with dementia (with increased general wellbeing as a result of doll therapy) is more likely to settle into a better quality of sleep, although this was poorly explored in the evidence. Interestingly, one study (Bisiani and Angus 2013) even identified better mobilisation of a resident (Mary, the resident living with a dementia observed in their single case study). This was attributed to a reduction in episodes of anxiety that manifested as hyperventilation and tremors (which had previously been so severe that they had caused falls).

Barriers to doll therapy

While there were a number of benefits associated with doll therapy, a number of challenges were also identified. According to this review, the therapeutic use of dolls for people living with dementia was approached in two main ways – either as an intervention or as a therapy. In the case of an intervention, which means dolls being offered to people for a set period of time, this was less common

(Cohen-Mansfield *et al.* 2010; Minshull 2009; Pezzati *et al.* 2014; Tamura *et al.* 2001). Naturally, these studies could not assess the long-term impact of dolls in the way that the other studies could. The therapeutic engagement of dolls was deemed as a 'therapy' when it was provided to people living with dementia over a longer period of time (e.g. from months to years). As a long-term 'therapy', healthcare professionals were not required to engage directly with doll therapy (i.e. people living with dementia used the dolls without direction) (Alander *et al.* 2013; Bisiani and Angus 2013; Ellingford *et al.* 2007; James *et al.* 2006; Mackenzie *et al.* 2006; Stephens *et al.* 2013). This was in contrast to the interventional studies, where healthcare professionals guided or led people living with dementia on how to use the dolls. These differing approaches raise questions about how best to implement doll therapy in practice.

Considering the person living with dementia, no studies were identified in this review that directly reported any limitations to doll therapy. However, some authors alluded to some potential problems associated with the use of dolls. While doll therapy has clear benefits associated with its use, its effect is not always long-term. Indeed, a few studies suggested that some people who engage with dolls appeared to lose interest over time (Stephens *et al.* 2013; Tamura *et al.* 2001). Ironically, while one of the key attributes of doll therapy was reduction in distressing behaviour, there were some instances where doll use actually caused distress (Alander *et al.* 2013; Bisiani and Angus 2013; James *et al.* 2006; Mackenzie *et al.* 2006; Stephens et al, 2013). In particular, those who engaged with the dolls could become possessive of their doll and refuse to be parted from it (James *et al.* 2006; Stephens *et al.* 2013). This possessive behaviour can manifest as either desirable, because the person living with dementia has forged a therapeutic attachment with her doll, or undesirable, because the person can become distressed if she is separated from her doll.

While these findings were not consistently reported, they are important nonetheless.

Healthcare professionals' attitudes were found to be a potential barrier to engagement with doll therapy (James *et al.* 2006; Mackenzie *et al.* 2006; Minshull 2009). In the study carried out by Mackenzie *et al.* (2006, p.442), they found, through use of questionnaires, that some people thought the use of dolls was 'babyish…demeaning…patronising…inappropriate'. These attitudes were observed in practice through Minshull's work, who noted that during her doll therapy intervention, 'nursing assistants were sniggering' (2009, p.37). Interestingly, the authors who identified staff scepticism as a potential issue appeared to correct this through education (Mackenzie *et al.* 2006; Minshull 2009). Administration of literature, information sessions and on-the job experience were shown to increase healthcare professionals' awareness and practice with doll therapy.

Of the 14 studies identified in the review, only 5 were explicit about their theoretical underpinnings (Alander *et al.* 2013; Bisiani and Angus 2013; Fraser and James 2008; Shin 2015; Stephens *et al.* 2013). Of those that were explicit about the use of theory, all of them chose to blend Bowlby's attachment theory (1969) with Kitwood's theory of personhood (1997). Stephens *et al.* (2013) were the only authors to use Winnicott's transitional object theory (1953). Interestingly the studies identified in this review that do underpin their research with theory are the more recent, which perhaps illuminates the emerging development of research into doll therapy. Undoubtedly an explicit theoretical foundation is important with regards to doll therapy because, as found in this review, health professionals may be resistive to using the therapy, and so making the case from a sound theoretical basis is important. (The theoretical underpinnings that have been applied to doll therapy in dementia care will be critically discussed in Chapter 3.)

The findings of these empirical studies have highlighted a number of potential benefits in the use of doll therapy for people living with dementia. In particular, the studies have associated therapeutic engagement with dolls as a means to promote the wellbeing of people living with dementia, particularly through improvements in activities of living. The empirical studies included in this review provide some insight to potential challenges associated with doll therapy, but in less depth when compared to its benefits. Limited professional awareness about appropriate use of the therapy, problems pertaining to doll ownership and negative pre-existing ideologies about the therapy appear to be the main challenges of the therapy, according to the literature review.

Table 2.1: Individual findings from empirical research

Author/ Year/ Country	Aim	Method	Sample	Key Findings
1 Tamura et al. (2001) Japan *Miyazaki*	To assess if dolls could be therapeutic for people with advanced dementia	• Following presentation of three dolls, by an occupational therapist (OT), people living with dementia were observed (by OT) • Results were categorised into four categories (no reaction, close observation, taking care of the doll or communication with other patients)	• 13 people living with dementia (3 male and 10 female) living in a long-term care facility • Average age of 90.2 (range 82–102) • All had Alzheimer's disease • Purposive sample (authors selected 13 residents with twilight syndrome (those living with dementia who experience higher amounts of distress in the late afternoon or early evening) from 40)	• People living with dementia in this study preferred the more 'realistic' baby doll – those that were 'made of silicon, which mimics the texture of a real baby' (p.117) • Most people living with dementia believed the dolls were real babies • People living with dementia who will engage with a doll will do so within around 90 seconds. The most common observed behaviours from engagement were: 'carrying while supporting the doll's neck, clasping the doll's hand, calling out to dolls' (p.115) • While there were brief accounts of men engaging with dolls, the phenomenon was mainly applicable to women

| 2 | Mackenzie et al. (2006) England *Newcastle* | Pilot study to examine the impact of the introduction of dolls on people living in a dementia care unit | • Dolls offered to all residents with dementia. If residents selected a doll, their interaction was monitored by staff over a 3–6 week period
• 5-item questionnaire for all care staff
• In addition, key workers of those who engaged with doll therapy were asked to complete a 14-item questionnaire. This sought to assess the impact of the doll on the person (i.e. level of activity, agitation and interactions with others) | • 37 people living with dementia offered a doll
• 14 people living with dementia (12 women and 2 men) used the doll
• Non-probability sample (all 37 residents were included in this study)
• 46 care staff completed 5-item questionnaire (96% response in care home 1 and 79% response in care home 2)
• 100% response to second questionnaire from 14 key workers
• Neither home employed 'qualified staff'(p.441) | • 14 dolls out of the 20 were used by residents. This represented 38% of the care unit population
• 35% of carers reported some problems with the dolls, namely, arguments between residents over ownership, residents trying to feed their dolls and dolls being misled' (p.442)
• In relation to initial impressions on doll therapy, 9 staff had either major/minor concerns, 16 were neutral and 21 were minor/majorly positive. In relation to concerns, quotes include 'thought it was babyish, totally demeaning, patronising, inappropriate and could confuse residents further' (p.442)
• Wellbeing of the people who used dolls was judged to be either a little better (30%) or much better (70%) by carers. In particular, staff perceived the dolls to be calming (p.443)
• Wellbeing increases were associated with the following: 'greater levels of interaction with staff, fellow residents, appeared happier, less agitated and more amenable to personal-care activities' (p.442) |

cont.

	Author/ Year/ Country	Aim	Method	Sample	Key Findings
3	James et al. (2006) England Newcastle	Following on from the Mackenzie et al. (2006) pilot study, the authors sought to examine how: 1) Doll therapy affected people living with dementia 2) If residents had preference of either a doll or teddy bear 3) If care staff could predict which residents would opt to engage with the dolls	• 15 dolls and 15 teddy bears were offered to people living with dementia in one care facility • 2 members of staff were selected by home manager to monitor residents prior to therapy: 1) They would complete a prediction sheet (i.e. to predict which residents would engage with the therapy) 2) They would complete an impact questionnaire (Likert scale) to access the therapy – the 5-point questionnaire used in the Mackenzie et al. (2006) pilot. These impact sheets were completed at weeks 1, 2, 4, 8 and 12 post-introduction of the toys	• 33 people living with dementia were offered a doll or teddy bear • 14 people living with dementia engaged with dolls (12 women and 2 men) • 2 members of staff were selected by care home manager	• Care staff only predicted with 56% accuracy which residents would use the doll. The 2 care staff members, however, were more accurate in relation to residents they felt would not use the doll (82% accuracy) • 14 residents out of 34 (41%) engaged with doll therapy • 13 out of 14 residents (93%) opted for a doll as opposed to a teddy bear when offered the choice • General wellbeing increase was noted for those using dolls in the form of 'activity, interaction, happiness' (p.1095). One resident referred to her doll by a name; one (a former GP) regularly examined the body of the doll. A group of women sat together with their dolls and interacted with one another – 'staff labelled these as the mothers group' (p.1095) • Some residents were noted to have obtained 'little, if any beneficial effects from doll usage' (p.1095). However, the authors go on to comment that doll therapy did not worsen the wellbeing of anyone with dementia during their study • One resident became possessive of her doll and would take other people's dolls, which caused some distress. Other examples of ownership problems were noted, despite all residents having their own personal dolls. Another challenge pertained to staff and relatives' opinions on dolls. One relative removed the doll from his mother, and some staff felt the therapy was demeaning

	Author	Aim	Method	Participants	Findings
4	Ellingford *et al.* (2007) England *Newcastle*	To examine the impact of doll therapy by retrospective analysis of case notes of residents before and after the introduction of dolls	Retrospective audit of residents' case notes, examining data over a 6-month period (3 months pre-doll and 3 months post-doll therapy)	66 people living with dementia from 4 care homes already using doll therapy (34 residents used doll therapy and 32 did not)	• 92% of the doll users were female • All those who used a doll showed 'significant improvement in all of the behavioural measures' (p.37)
5	Fraser and James (2008) England *Newcastle*	To develop an understanding of why doll therapy improves the wellbeing of some people living with dementia	2 semi-structured interviews with 8 health professionals First interview was exploratory while the second was designed to receive feedback on a model the authors constructed based on the first round of interviews	8 health professionals (included 2 psychologists, 2 nurses, 2 care assistants, 1 psychiatrist and 1 OT)	• Participants perceived that doll therapy could meet a number of individual needs for people living with dementia, which included 'attachment, comfort, inclusion, activity, communication, interaction, identity and fantasy' (p.56) • In relation to attachment, 'when residents move into a care home, they often lose figures and/or objects of meaningful attachment, such as family members [dolls could offer support this emerging need]' (p.56) • In relation to communication, healthcare professionals suggested that common conversation could be shared between the health professional and the person with dementia

cont.

	Author/ Year/ Country	Aim	Method	Sample	Key Findings
6	Minshull (2009) Scotland *Edinburgh*	To identify whether doll therapy improved wellbeing for people living with dementia	• Unstructured doll therapy sessions carried out on a hospital ward by an OT once a week for one month • The Bradford Dementia Group Wellbeing Profiling Tool (2002) was used to assess the reactions of people pre/post-doll therapy • Wellbeing profiling was carried out by the author and verified by a student OT	• 9 people living with dementia engaged with dolls along with an unspecified number of nursing professionals	• For the 9 people engaging in doll therapy, there was a notable increase in the wellbeing of 7 • The author observed that healthcare staff appeared to naturally play with the doll, 'bouncing it on my knee while reminiscing with a patient' (p.37) • Healthcare staff commented that prior education on doll therapy was extremely limited, and additional reading material, provided by the authors prior to the study, was very beneficial • Post-study, the author states that the doll therapy sessions have continued, and that the department has purchased a pram in order to further doll activities
7	Cohen-Mansfield *et al.* (2010) USA *Maryland*	• To examine the impact of different stimuli on people living with dementia • While not explicitly based on doll therapy, this study did post findings on the phenomenon	Each person was presented with 23 predetermined different engagement stimuli (e.g. life-like baby doll, a robotic animal, a real baby, a real dog, a magazine, a ball etc.)	• 193 people living with dementia residing in 7 care homes • Average age of 86 • (151 female, 42 male)	• With specific attention to the phenomenon of doll therapy, residents who chose to engage with dolls were considerably more likely to spend longer with life-like dolls • The authors also found that residents preferred dolls as opposed to animal-shaped toys

8	Green et al. (2011) USA *Chicago*	To determine the effects of doll therapy on geriatric patients related to PRN (pro re nata, medications administered as necessary or as a result of symptoms) prescriptions of Haloperidol	Staff observations were recorded in a log book	• All patients admitted to the 21 bed gero-psychiatric unit over a period of 3 months • (115 patients, 72 women, 43 men) • Mean age of 69 • 39% of these participants had a clinical diagnosis of dementia	The authors found that people engaging in doll therapy were more likely to receive less PRN Haloperidol prescriptions as opposed to those who didn't
9	Stephens et al. (2013) England *Bristol*	To explore the relationship people living with dementia have with physical objects using focused ethnography	• 21 residents and the staff of a care home were observed over a 2-month period • 30 hours of observation were completed over a 2-month period	21 people living with dementia and 27 staff members	• A resident with dementia was observed carrying a plastic doll in the style of a young baby, 'she would not let go of it, and would become distressed if she thought it was being taken' (p.701). Attachment was considered as a need that could be met through dolls • In another observation, one resident would not relinquish her doll even when it needed to be washed. Even when the family brought a second doll, the resident would not engage in the same way with the substitute • The authors found that the dolls should seem real, or have warmth, texture, or some quality that shows them to have 'reality'. This realism would promote a more authentic experience (i.e. because the doll was thought to be a baby)

cont.

	Author/ Year/ Country	Aim	Method	Sample	Key Findings
10	Bisiani and Angus (2013) Australia *Melbourne*	To examine the therapeutic effect of a life-like baby doll on a person living with dementia	Observation alongside Aged Care Funding Instrument (ACFI) to evaluate wellbeing	Case study of 1 female participant with moderately advanced Alzheimer's disease	• Prior to doll therapy, Mary was socially withdrawn and did not communicate with many people, she wandered and became easily distressed. Following the introduction of a doll, these behaviours were noted to have decreased: 'Reduction in appearance of anxiety, panic, tremors, hyperventilation and searching' (p.456) • 'Improvement in dining experience, social interaction with staff and other residents, improved self-esteem as Mary was so proud to be the "one" with the doll' (p.457)
11	Alander *et al.* (2013) England *Newcastle*	To understand how people in care, doll users and non-doll users make sense of a doll in their setting	Focus group interview with 5 participants and semi-structured interviews with 11	• 16 participants (11 of which had dementia, 4 were actively using dolls) • 2 doll users were male and 2 were female	• Both doll users and non-doll users believed that a doll represented a sense of ownership, which promoted a sense of control • It also filled people with a sense of pride. One doll user remarked, 'I'm bringing them up marvellous you see' (p.5) • Almost all participants believed engagement with a doll gave a sense of purpose and provided an activity to keep the person occupied. Some participants perceived that this would protect doll users from becoming lonely, bored or isolated • Dolls could promote a sense of attachment or bonding as evidenced by 'carrying, feeding, bathing, dressing' (p.6)

12	Pezzati *et al.* (2014) Italy *Como*	To measure if doll therapy could preserve or promote attachment in people with dementia	• Video observation by research team of 10 individual sessions per person. 5 sessions with a doll and 5 with a colourful soft rubber foam cube • 50% of people had been exposed to doll therapy before and 50% had not	• 10 people living with dementia in a care home • (9 females and 1 male) • Age range 72–92	• Both groups (people who had previously engaged with doll therapy and people who had never engaged with doll therapy) showed greater levels of caregiving behaviour when engaging with a doll • People who used doll therapy were more likely to lose interest in the foam cube before the doll
13	Braden and Gaspar (2014) USA *Toledo*	To measure the impact of doll therapy on residents at a dementia care centre	Reported outcome measurement of happiness, activity, interaction, ease of personal care and anxiety by nursing staff	• 16 women living with dementia • Age range 60–94	• There was generally an improvement in happiness, level of activity, interaction and ease of personal care. However, results were less dramatic than other studies • There was no statistically significant data across the self-reported domains
14	Shin (2015) South Korea *Seoul*	To examine if doll therapy could positively impact the wellbeing of people living with dementia in a care home	Questionnaire administered to nursing staff about changes in mood, behaviour, social interaction and episodes of distress	51 people living with dementia in a care home	Linear regression demonstrated statistically significant differences in aggression, obsessive behaviours, wandering, negative verbalisation, negative mood and negative physical appearance after introduction of the doll therapy intervention. Interactions with other individuals also increased over time

Critical discussion

There is evidence in the literature to suggest that the use of dolls can provide therapeutic gains for some people living with dementia. The empirical evidence appears to provide limited direction on how best to use doll therapy, with a clear division as to whether dolls should be used as an intervention or as a therapy, and also whether this should be in a nursing home facility or on a hospital ward. The only guidelines that exist were reported by the authors from the Newcastle Challenging Behaviour Team (NCBT) (Mackenzie *et al.* 2006), who admittedly are best placed to provide these, given that they have conducted 5 of the 14 empirical studies in this area (Alander *et al.* 2013; Ellingford *et al.* 2007; Fraser and James 2008; James *et al.* 2006; Mackenzie *et al.* 2006). Despite their expertise and enterprising work, there are obvious questions pertaining to the transferability of doll therapy to other clinical settings. Ostensibly, then, many healthcare professionals consider doll therapy controversial or even contentious (Mitchell 2014).

The use of doll therapy in clinical practice is not automatically right or wrong, but if it is practised or used in a meaningful way, it has the potential to be truly person-centred. Person-centred care is underpinned by respect, understanding and an enablement of practices that facilitate self-determination (McCormack *et al.* 2010a, 2010b). Due to the paucity of literature on doll therapy it is important that knowledge about appropriate practices and underpinning theory is delivered effectively. As demonstrated in this review, one of the key challenges to doll therapy was preconceptions or education of healthcare professionals who are key in enablement of the therapy. The learning culture of a clinical environment is particularly important, and McCormack, Dewing and McCance (2011) assert that any sustained learning will only occur in a supportive context.

The application of doll therapy to the person-centred nursing (PCN) framework, developed by McCormack and McCance (2006, 2010) from their previous work on person-centred practice with older people (McCormack 2003), and the experience of caring in nursing (McCance 2006), is particularly useful when considering the contents of this review. McCormack and McCance's (2010) PCN framework comprises four constructs: pre-requisites, the care environment, person-centred processes and outcomes (McCance *et al.* 2011; McCormack and McCance 2010; McCormack *et al.* 2010a, 2010b, 2012). The PCN framework can be an effective tool for nurses to use in the practice of doll therapy, and is considered as follows:

- *Pre-requisites:* This focuses on the nurse's attributes, which should include professional competence, well-developed interpersonal skills and commitment to their role. When considering doll therapy, engagement with dolls can only work if the nurse facilitates this. This review has demonstrated that those living with dementia who are likely to glean benefits from doll therapy must be enabled or empowered by others. As all of these studies were conducted in clinical settings, this enablement is likely to be facilitated by a nurse.

- *Care environment:* This focuses on the context in which care is delivered, and should provide organisational systems that are supportive, facilitate a sharing of power between the person and nurse, and there is potential for innovation and risk-taking. Building on the previous construct, the care environment should allow nurses to engage with doll therapy. Given the limited, but encouraging, evidence that is on offer, doll therapy might be considered an innovative approach for some living with dementia. For those practitioners who are less convinced, it may represent an opportunity of a balanced risk, given the potential benefits for the person living with dementia.

- *Person-centred processes:* This focuses on delivering care through a range of therapeutic avenues that incorporate the person's (patient's) beliefs, values, shared decision-making and the provision of physical care. This construct is also underpinned by sympathetic presence. As demonstrated, doll therapy can facilitate and support person-centred processes because of the potential for improvement in many facets of daily living activities identified in this review.

- *Outcomes:* This is the central component of the PCN model, and should include outcomes such as satisfaction with care, involvement in care, increased wellbeing and promotion of the therapeutic environment. Doll therapy has the potential to enhance meaningful engagement with people who are living with dementia, and in addition, it has the ability to connect with the person's innate caring quality (i.e. caring for a baby).

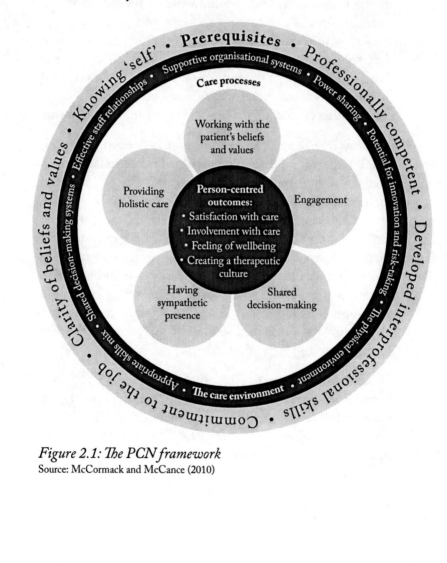

Figure 2.1: The PCN framework
Source: McCormack and McCance (2010)

Why does doll therapy work in dementia care?

Attachment and transitional objects

It has been suggested that the reason doll therapy works so well in dementia care is because of the benefits that are associated with a person's attachment needs. Many have attributed John Bowlby's work on attachment theory (Bowlby 1969) as the central rationale as to why doll therapy has the potential to be therapeutic for people living with dementia (Mitchell and O'Donnell 2013; Stephens *et al.* 2013). Attachment has long been identified as a key psychological need for people living with dementia due to the new challenges, anxiety and uncertainties that are faced as a result of the advancing disease (Kitwood 1997; Miesen 1993). It is noteworthy that Bowlby's conceptual work on attachment theory was actually originally intended for child populations and not for people living with dementia (Bowlby 1969) – Bere Miesen (1993) first applied the principles of attachment theory to people living with dementia. Miesen believed that fixating on one's parents, or the way some people living with dementia continually search for their parents, is an expression of an attachment need. This searching behaviour was perhaps evidence that the person living with dementia was in an unknown, insecure environment, and sought reunion with a family in order to feel safe. If attachment needs are not met in times of anxiety or uncertainty, that person may see her level of wellbeing diminish, and this, in turn, leads to distress (Kitwood 1997; Miesen 1993).

With attention to the 'doll', the theoretical work of Winnicott (1953) is also used (Bisiani and Angus 2013; Mitchell and O'Donnell 2013). Winnicott (1953), again basing his psychological theory on child populations, noted that a 'transitional object' is sometimes used by children when they are separated from their parents as it enables them to feel a greater level of security in an uncertain environment (Loboprabhu, Molinari and Lomax 2007). Winnicott (1953) suggested that children used soft toys, blankets or even repetitive behaviours or phrases as a transitional object during times of uncertainty. From the work of Bowlby (1969), Miesen (1993) and Winnicott (1953), some theory has emerged that can be useful at describing how doll therapy can work with people living with dementia.

Emerging theory from the empirical evidence

As alluded to, there have been some scant theoretical underpinnings as to how doll therapy can enhance the wellbeing of people living with dementia based on the theories of attachment and person-centred care. Two studies identified in this review have produced comprehensive explanatory models based on grounded theory methods that are significant in relation to the emerging theory on doll therapy (Alander *et al.* 2013; Fraser and James 2008). Fraser and James (2008) developed a model, based on empirical investigation, to assist practitioners in understanding the rationale for improvement in wellbeing for people living with a dementia who engage with dolls. They acknowledged the importance of attachment in their model, but, importantly, recognised that there were a number of other equally pivotal factors including inclusion, comfort and identity. These factors directly correspond with what Kitwood determined were the fundamental needs of the person with dementia (Kitwood 1997). In addition to these factors, which correspond directly to previous theory on doll therapy, Fraser and James (2008) reported emerging factors that relate to activity, innate drivers and memories. Doll therapy could offer an opportunity for people living with a dementia to engage in meaningful activity, and as a result provide those living with a dementia with a sense of purpose (examples of this may include nursing, feeding, dressing or singing to the doll).

On innate drivers, Fraser and James (2008) found that participants believed that people engaging with dolls were responding to instinct-like behaviours, for example, the innate wish to engage in social contact. Through grounded theory analyses it was also suggested that doll therapy could evoke pleasurable memories for the person living with dementia. Alander, Prescott and James (2013) used grounded theory to explore older adults' views and experiences of doll therapy. This ultimately supplements Fraser and James' (2008) work, which drew on a healthcare professional group. Alander *et al.* (2013) found that there were a number of intrapersonal features that directly influenced the wellbeing of people living with dementia, and these included ownership of a doll, purpose, role and attachment. In addition to these intrapersonal features, Alander *et al.* (2013) found that there were also a number of external interpersonal factors that could promote a person's wellbeing, and these included companionship, communication with others and greater inclusion. Interestingly Alander *et al.* (2013) note that the majority of older adults involved in this study considered that intra/interpersonal factors were more likely to outweigh any practical or ethical concerns.

In addition to the two studies that sought to generate theory (Alander *et al.* 2013; Fraser and James 2008), only two other studies identified in this review made explicit reference to their theoretical underpinnings (Bisiani and Angus 2013; Stephens *et al.* 2013). These drew on Bowlby's attachment theory (1969) and Kitwood's theory of personhood (1997). Stephens *et al.* (2013) also used Winnicott's transitional object theory (1953). Interestingly, the studies identified in this review that do underpin their research with theory are the more recent, which perhaps highlights the emerging development of research into doll therapy. Undoubtedly an explicit theoretical foundation is important with regards to doll therapy because, as found in this review, healthcare professionals may be resistive to using the therapy, and therefore it is important to make the case from a sound theoretical basis.

Limitations of the review

One factor that was unclear from the empirical studies included in this review was the staging of dementia and the associated benefits from doll therapy. When considering the illness trajectory associated with dementia (Lunney *et al.* 2003; Murtagh, Preston and Higginson 2004; WHO 2004), there is no obvious stage (e.g. in early or late dementia) where engagement with dolls is the most therapeutic. That being stated, given the nature of the findings, it is probably a therapy that is most used by people in the middle to late stages of the illness.

Another limitation identified through this review pertains to the theoretical underpinnings of doll therapy for people living with dementia. From the review, there were inconsistent references to how doll therapy has the potential to enhance the wellbeing of those living with dementia. Those studies that did opted to use theory based on attachment and personhood. This is understandable given the paucity of research in this area.

Conclusion

The number of people living with dementia who are benefiting from therapeutic engagement with dolls is increasing. While empirical investigation has been limited, there are a number of encouraging results as well as many anecdotal accounts of its success. The results of doll therapy are unique to the person, and so it is impossible to predict what benefits a person living with dementia will have, if any, when engaging with a doll, but this review suggests improvements in overall communication, engagement with others, dietary intake and general wellbeing. However, despite the growing evidence of potential benefits to people living with dementia, doll therapy is still broached with caution by some. The main barrier to doll therapy appears to due to pre-existing ideas from healthcare professionals, who are crucial in its enablement. While the PCN framework offers a very useful structured approach to facilitating doll therapy in a person-centred way, the paucity of high-quality empirical evidence must still be acknowledged. There is a pressing need for further empirical study so healthcare professionals can be provided with greater evidence for the use of dolls in clinical practice.

Chapter 3

Doll Therapy and Dementia Care through Kitwood's Ideas

Gary Mitchell and Jan Dewing

While there is promising evidence that supports the use of dolls in dementia care, some practitioners, care partners and commentators still believe that doll therapy is controversial. This chapter presents an overview of the concept of person-centred care through the lens of the key ideas developed by Professor Tom Kitwood. Kitwood's theory on person-centred care in dementia forms the bedrock for a number of models for optimising the delivery of person-centred care, and is considered a seminal work as it pertains to person-centred dementia care. Two of Kitwood's ideas, namely, malignant social psychology and positive person work, are explored throughout this chapter, and applied to the practice of doll therapy in dementia care.

Background

The concept of person-centred care has been around for some time, and although associated with it, it predates the work of Carl Rogers over a half-century ago (Rogers 1961). The term 'person-centred care' refers to an approach to care that places the person at the centre of their own care in certain ways. In other words, the person is supported by healthcare professionals to identify what matters to him, to contribute to his own care, for example, making shared decisions about treatment and how he wants care provided through two-way communication underpinned by mutual respect between the person offering care and the person receiving care, and to contribute to evaluation of that care. Generally, person-centred care recognises the importance of the whole person and goes far beyond simply responding to or supporting medical management of biomedical disease, as it gives consideration to the person's values and aspirations, psychological, social and spiritual care (McCormack and McCance 2010). Person-centred care therefore prioritises dignity and respect and tends to be focused on a person's fundamental human rights (Perez-Merino 2014; Steenbergen *et al.* 2013). Fundamentally, person-centred care is underpinned by what we understand a person to be and what matters to people in his life, especially when he is unwell or ill, and reappraise his life in some way.

Personhood

'Personhood' is the term generally used to describe the essential attributes of being a person. When our personhood is 'full' we feel more like a person, more like ourselves. The sorts of things that matter to each of us about being a person might be remarkably similar, and yet at the same time, we might each have some different attributes (Dewing 2008). *Defining personhood* is a controversial topic in philosophy and law, and is closely bound to political concepts of citizenship, equality and liberty. For several centuries (Locke 1997), our sense of personhood has been, and still is, largely influenced by three characteristics: rationality, self-awareness and the linkage of our self-awareness and rationality with memory. We tend to admire and perhaps be in awe of those who excel in these attributes, and we exclude or (overly) protect those who are extremely deficient in the same attributes. No matter how carefully philosophers have tried to define personhood, the result has tended to be that some human beings are excluded from the status of being a person. Those of us lacking in cognitive abilities are one of the groups of human beings who more easily become excluded from being rewarded by society as a person and the entitlement of rights that accompanies being a person, for example, the right to freedom of movement and to have a private life and the right to give consent.

Moving into the dementia care field, Kitwood defines personhood as 'a standing or a status that is bestowed on one human being, by another in the context of relationship and social being' (Kitwood 1997, p.8). Although this definition is flawed in several ways, it is useful to keep in mind that Kitwood regards personhood as sacred and unique. Further, he argues that people with dementia have an absolute value (however advanced the dementia), requiring others 'to treat each other with deep respect' (Kitwood 1997, p.8). People with dementia used to be regarded as lesser or even non-persons when it came to caregiving. This meant that that many fundamental human needs (see Figure 3.1 on page 57) were not provided or were at worst deliberately removed. This resulted in feelings of emptiness, sadness, loneliness, feeling devalued and ultimately feeling completely unloved. Consequently, the person with dementia would communicate these feelings through behaviours of distress, which were often labelled as challenging behaviours, and even the person was labelled as challenging. When the person with dementia was offered ways of meeting his fundamental human needs, this led to feelings of value, self-worth, attachment, occupation and being loved or being able to love another (see Figure 3.1 on page 57).

Malignant social psychology and positive person work

We are now going to build on Kitwood's ideas a little more to show how doll therapy can be understood against the backdrop of personhood. Professor Tom Kitwood was a major influence in the field of dementia care as his work paved the way for numerous models of person-centred care that are used in dementia care today (Kitwood 1993, 1995, 1997). Kitwood's interpretation of personhood in dementia care formed the basis for two sets of ideas: malignant social psychology (and the associated Illbeing and Wellbeing Scale) and positive person work (Kitwood 1997). These seminal theories are still used today across medicine, nursing and allied health to demonstrate the fundamentals of person-centred caring with people living with dementia. In short, malignant social psychology tells us about the ways in which the personhood of people living with dementia can be reduced in a caring relationship or in a care setting. This leads to and perpetuates feelings of illbeing, while positive person work leads to feelings of wellbeing and can enhance the personhood of people living with dementia. Supporting a person living with dementia to fulfil his personhood is a key goal of person-centred care.

From his research, Kitwood (1997) identified a number of barriers in practice and care settings that actually serve to undermine the personhood of people living with dementia. He described these barriers as malignant social psychology. As will be explored in the next section of this chapter, malignant social psychology is a group of often quite simple behaviours, actions or non-actions that serve to undermine the personhood of those living with dementia. These behaviours are often usually as a result of healthcare workers or care partners who lack specialist dementia education, and are usually not purposeful or malicious.

Kitwood (1997) illustrated these malignant behaviours and actions to help practitioners, and indeed care partners, see when they were happening, so they could then avoid them in order to enhance the experiences of those living with dementia in care. Thus, it is possible to reduce the range of malignant behaviours or actions and to reduce the severity of their impact on the person with dementia. We can imagine how one person with dementia dependent on others in a number of ways can, over time, have his personhood whittled away by being ignored, by being bored and unoccupied, by repeatedly being told he shouldn't do something or by being made to feel he can't accomplish a task.

In addition to providing an overview of behaviours that would diminish the personhood of those living with dementia, Kitwood recognised that enhancing personhood wasn't just about the absence of malignant social psychology; personhood needed nurturing. So he also described a number of behaviours or actions that would enhance the personhood of people living with dementia, and called this positive person work. While the theories of malignant social psychology and positive person work assist practitioners in operationalising person-centred practices every day and in every care encounter, we should always note that person-centred care is about a bigger picture – the main psychological needs of people living with dementia, as shown in Figure 3.1. Kitwood (1997) theorised that the needs of attachment, inclusion, occupation, identity and comfort are present in all human beings, and that for those living with dementia, these needs were likely to be heightened. This is because people living with dementia are perhaps more vulnerable and less likely to be able to take action for themselves to satisfy these needs as their condition progresses (Kitwood 1997).

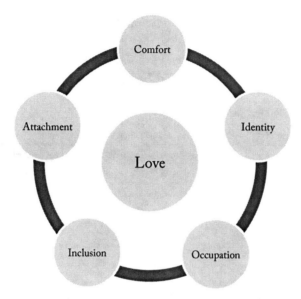

Figure 3.1: Psychological needs of people living with dementia

It is possible to see how doll therapy could be used to enhance these core human needs. However, when used with a poor understanding about its overall purpose or in a less than positive way, practitioners or care partners may also be introducing aspects of malignant social psychology and undermining personhood.

To summarise, comfort relates to the feeling of trust that comes from others, attachment is linked to security and finding familiarity in unusual places, inclusion is about being involved in the lives of others, occupation pertains to being involved in the processes of normal life and identity is what distinguishes that person from others and as such makes him unique (Kitwood 1997). Whether these psychological needs are met, and subsequently, if personhood is maintained or enhanced, is in large part related to the care staff/ care environment, and whether behaviour corresponds more with the malignant social psychology or the positive person work model (Mitchell and Agnelli 2015b).

Malignant social psychology

As illustrated, malignant social psychology describes a range of behaviours or actions and non-actions that undermine the personhood of those living with dementia (Kitwood 1997). Kitwood (1997), based on his own observations carried out in practice, went on to describe a number of ways that the personhood of people living with a dementia could be undermined across all care settings. Undoubtedly, recurring episodes of malignant social psychology undermine the personhood of individuals living with dementia. These are described in Table 3.1.

Table 3.1: Malignant social psychology

Malignancies	Definition
Treachery	Using deception in order to distract or manipulate behaviour
Disempowerment	Not allowing or enabling a person to use the abilities he still has
Infantilisation	Treating the person like a child
Intimidation	Causing the person to feel fearful as a result of threat or physical power
Labelling	Referring to people inappropriately, e.g. 'elderly mentally infirm'
Stigmatisation	Treating the person as if he were an outcast
Outpacing	Providing information or choices too quickly, thus potentially making information difficult to understand
Invalidation	Not acknowledging the reality of the person
Banishment	Excluding the person either physically or emotionally
Objectification	Treating the person as an object, e.g. during washing/dressing
Ignoring	Conversing with others in the presence of the person as if he is not present
Imposition	Forcing the person to do something
Withholding	Failing to provide attention or meet an obvious need
Accusation	Blaming a person for his misunderstanding or inability
Disruption	Suddenly disturbing a person and interrupting his activity/ thoughts
Mockery	Making fun or joking at the expense of the person
Disparagement	Telling the person that he is worthless

Source: Adapted from Kitwood (1997); Mitchell and Agnelli (2015b)

Kitwood (1997) believed that the main cause of malignant social psychology was, and probably still is, because people living with dementia were not always encouraged to be visible or acknowledged in society, and that others had a poor understanding of dementia. Hence, at this time, a lot of effort is being put into creating wide-scale dementia awareness.

Positive person work

Malignant social psychology is contrasted with positive person work. Unlike the former, positive person work is about enhancing the wellbeing of people living with dementia by fulfilling the psychological needs of those living with dementia that Kitwood identified, shown in Figure 3.1. Similarly to malignant social psychology, Kitwood identified a number of behaviours or actions that are needed to form the basis of dementia care. These are detailed in Table 3.2.

Kitwood's work and its application to doll therapy

Tom Kitwood died in 1998, before the first empirical study on the use of doll therapy took place in 2001 (Tamura *et al.* 2001). As a result, he was not able to critically evaluate the therapeutic use of dolls in dementia care. Given the importance of Kitwood's work, it is hardly surprising that his theories on malignant social psychology and positive person work have been interpreted by scholars, researchers and clinicians over the years (Mitchell and Templeton 2014), and are drawn on here to help us understand how doll therapy can contribute to wellbeing and to enhancing personhood. In Chapter 6 the therapeutic use of dolls will be considered within a bioethical context with some reference to Tom Kitwood's work. In order to show how Kitwood's theories have been interpreted with respect to doll therapy in dementia care, there now follows a hypothetical scenario, which is then critically analysed.

Table 3.2: Positive person work

Positive person work	Definition
Recognition	A person who is recognised by name and acknowledged as a person with unique thoughts, feelings and preferences, e.g. greeting a person by his preferred name
Negotiation	Facilitated through consultation with the person about his preferences in care and his daily life. Where possible he is supported to be involved in the decision-making process, e.g. serving a resident food that he enjoys
Collaboration	Partnership between healthcare professional and the person in order to carry out an activity or task, e.g. having a bath or getting dressed in ways that are comfortable for the person
Play	The provision of appropriate activity and enablement of self-expression, e.g. rolling a ball, sharing a joke or playing a game
Giving	Accepting whatever kindness the person with dementia gives, e.g. the person with dementia may want to give a nurse a flower from the garden
Timilation	A form of interaction, like aromatherapy, which is sensual
Celebration	Not just during celebratory occasions, like birthdays or anniversaries, but the person should see his achievements celebrated, e.g. joining the person who is happy and celebrating, irrespective of the reason, by clapping, whistling, singing or smiling
Relaxation	Low level of intensity and recognition that some people may like to relax in solitude, e.g. listening to music or spending time in the garden
Validation	Connected to Feil's work, this is about accepting the reality of another even if it is as the result of hallucinations or misperceptions
Holding	To provide a safe psychological space or environment so as to enable people to truly express themselves, e.g. if a person with dementia is experiencing distress, do not isolate him, stay beside him and validate his experiences without trying to stop or ignore him
Creation	Encouraging the person to be creative as this can be therapeutic, e.g. spontaneous singing or dancing, or horticultural therapy
Facilitation	Enabling the person to do what otherwise he would be unable to do. This is similar to collaboration, e.g. accompanying a person to go for a walk outside of the unit

Source: Adapted from Kitwood (1997); Mitchell and Agnelli (2015b)

Scenario

Clara is an older woman who lives with dementia in a care home. She was diagnosed with Alzheimer's disease, the most common type of dementia, five years ago. Clara's dementia has progressed, and she now needs assistance with a number of activities of daily living in relation to eating and drinking, elimination, washing and dressing, communication and mobilisation. Clara has been experiencing more episodes of distress as her condition progresses, and recently found comfort in an empathy doll that the care staff provided. Clara calls her doll 'Tom', and believes that he is a living baby that she cares for. Clara likes to feed Tom, put Tom to bed and hold Tom throughout the day.

Scenario analysis: Using the lens of malignant social psychology

The most common negative perception of doll therapy often centres on what Kitwood termed 'infantilisation'. This is because infantilisation is about treating people with dementia like they are children. Family, care partners, or indeed experienced care staff, may perceive providing a doll to Clara as treating people with dementia like children – children have dolls. This is not always the case, of course. Many adults have fluffy animals and similar objects; some continue to sleep and play with them too. Infantilisation has the potential to perpetuate the stigma associated with dementia care and support erroneous claims that Clara is, in some way, now an outcast of society because her behaviour is not considered 'normal'. As noted, stigmatisation was another strand of malignant social psychology that could undermine the personhood of those living with dementia.

As also noted in the review of the empirical evidence detailed in Chapter 2, one of the main challenges of doll therapy is a limited knowledge base among lay people and healthcare workers. Without knowledge of the therapeutic benefits of doll therapy, there is the potential that these individuals may wrongly label the person living with dementia as child-like because he uses a doll or perhaps even mock their use. If Clara's family, care staff, or even other visitors to the care home are not informed about the rationale behind doll therapy, they may even privately use terminology that is demeaning, for example referring to Clara as infantile or 'babyish'. They may also have negative views about the care team for using dolls. Kitwood theorised that mockery and labelling were also two concepts of malignant social psychology.

Perhaps less common, but definitely applicable, interpretations of malignant social psychology in doll therapy pertain to imposition, treachery and disempowerment. These three traits relate to using doll therapy in practice. Imposition is about forcing a person living with dementia to do something that they may not want to, for example, engaging in doll therapy. While this does not apply to Clara, because she enjoys engaging with dolls, it may be applicable if practitioners attempt to replicate the therapy on other residents within the care home that Clara lives in. As noted throughout this book, doll therapy is not for everybody, and there is no way to ascertain if someone will derive therapeutic benefit or not. In other words, if a person chooses not to engage with a doll, this should be noted as his preference, and he should not be forced to do so. Treachery is about using deception to manipulate a person's behaviour. It has been suggested, both in the anecdotal and empirical evidence base, that if a person living with dementia believes his doll is alive and calls it by a certain name, then family, care partners and healthcare workers should do the same. In other words, family, care staff and any visitors who come into contact with Clara should refer to her doll as 'Tom' because that is what she has named it. In addition, these practitioners should not tell or suggest that Tom is not living or a doll. This may be interpreted as treachery because the literature clearly recommends that going along with a person is appropriate on these occasions, even though it is not strictly truthful. Finally, disempowerment, which is not allowing the person living with dementia to use the abilities he still has, is noteworthy because, as described earlier in this book, some people living with dementia who engage with dolls can become over-reliant on their use, and when the doll is removed, either purposively or accidentally, he is not able to function as well without it.

Scenario analysis: Using the lens of positive person work

While malignant social psychology has been used as a lens to disparage therapeutic engagement with dolls in dementia care, the opposite is true of positive person work that has been used as a lens to celebrate the contribution that doll therapy can make for some people living with dementia.

Although some believe that doll therapy has the potential to be infantile and increase the possible stigma associated with the dementia diseases, Kitwood advocated that play and creation were important facets of good dementia care. He saw play as an age-appropriate activity that would enable self-expression, associated with numerous activities, one of which could be doll therapy. Kitwood also postulated that people living with dementia should be encouraged to be creative because it could be therapeutic and enhance the personhood of that individual. In Clara's case, her engagement with a doll enables her to be creative, as noted by the variety of ways she garners therapeutic benefit from her doll Tom, for example, helping to feed the doll or putting the doll to bed.

Unsurprisingly, therapeutic engagement with dolls can also be mapped across to another key part of positive person work, relaxation. This invariably leads to people experiencing less episodes of distress as they are encouraged to enjoy activities that are calm or relaxing. In Clara's case, and indeed in many others identified in the anecdotal and empirical literature, doll therapy is commonly associated with reducing episodes of distress that people living with dementia experience.

Another key component of positive person work, which is paramount when considering doll therapy, is validation. Kitwood believed that it was optimum practice for care workers, care partners and family to recognise that people living with dementia often experience an altered reality to others due to the manifestations of the dementia diseases. As noted, Clara believes her doll is a living baby called Tom. While some may consider going along with this reality as treachery, it is actually considered as validation, which is a key aspect of positive person work. Validation, which originated from Feil's work (1993), is considered to be something that only people with true empathy and understanding can deliver in dementia care.

Finally, facilitation should also be considered. In other words, people living with dementia should be enabled to do what they otherwise would not be able to do. In Clara's case, she has been facilitated to engage in doll therapy with good result. In addition, it was also noted in the empirical review of the literature in Chapter 2 that many living with dementia who engage with doll therapy actually see improvements in some of their aspects of daily living – doll therapy has been shown to facilitate some people living with dementia to do what they previously could not do.

Conclusion

It is beyond the scope of this chapter to consider a variety of person-centred care models that are currently being effectively used in dementia care, for example, the VIPS model (Brooker 2007), Nolan *et al.*'s senses framework (2006) and McCormack and McCance's person-centred practice framework (2006, 2010). Incidentally, McCormack and McCance's framework was used in interpreting the empirical evidence in Chapter 2. While these person-centred care theories have developed person-centred practices since Kitwood's original work (1993, 1995, 1997), dementia care education often begins with Tom Kitwood's original work. From personal experience, Kitwood's work is still often favoured by healthcare professionals in dementia care as it provides an overview of clinical practice that is either advocated (positive person work) or discouraged (malignant social psychology).

The key point to make is that practitioners can be much clearer and more systematic about the bigger picture of contributing to enhancing personhood when they draw on models, as they tend to offer a structure for thinking what is the best thing to do for the person with dementia, how different aspects of care relate to each other, and to enhancing personhood.

To summarise, the importance of person-centred care is without question, and it is positive to note that its influence on dementia care has been evolving since Kitwood's death. Healthcare professionals have a key responsibility in leading and disseminating best practice, and Kitwood's work (1997) has often provided a good starting point as it is provides an understandable direction for practitioners and indeed care partners in relation to what enhances personhood (positive person work) and what diminishes personhood (malignant social psychology).

The underpinning ethos of Kitwood's core ideas and indeed all theory on person-centred care is that all people are equal regardless of cognitive ability. This chapter illustrates that the therapeutic use of dolls in dementia care can benefit from being viewed through a theoretical lens. Theoretical ideas can provide an additional driver for implementing better care. In this situation, the challenge for practitioners and care partners is to enable delivery of doll therapy so that it is evidenced and seen by others to contribute to positive person work as opposed to malignant social psychology.

Tom Kitwood's work was pioneering within dementia care. His work on malignant social psychology and positive person work is still used today to educate practitioners about what enables and what prevents delivery of optimum levels of person-centred dementia care. Doll therapy in dementia care has a number of critics who appear to be grounded within the theoretical evidence base of Kitwood's malignant social psychology. It is important to acknowledge these because these are usually as a result of poor education in relation to doll therapy. When considering both the anecdotal and empirical evidence on offer, the therapeutic effect of engagement with dolls is more akin to the positive person work that Kitwood theorised. It is a challenge for healthcare workers, who can access the evidence on doll therapy, to provide education on doll therapy to co-workers, the multidisciplinary team, family members and care partners. Doll therapy in dementia care remains controversial, and it is helpful to have a balanced interpretation of the phenomenon through the lenses of Kitwood's work, and indeed person-centred care on the whole.

Chapter 4

The Ethics of Doll Therapy[1]

Gary Mitchell and Michelle Templeton

Thus far consideration has been given to the therapeutic use of dolls in dementia care in relation to the therapy itself, the available empirical evidence on its effectiveness in practice, and the theory behind why it can work. This chapter provides an overview of the ethical considerations of the topic. In short, doll therapy may be deemed controversial by some because giving a doll to a person living with dementia can be perceived as childish, and thus may perpetuate the stigma associated with the dementia diseases. Others may support doll therapy because of its positive impact on the lives of some people living with dementia.

To date, the use of dolls as a therapy in dementia care has been considered only/mainly in relation to the potential therapeutic benefits. As yet, understandings about the ethical, theoretical and practical application of its use are lacking. In this chapter, the authors seek to provide an overview of the ethical issues underpinning the topic, by discussing each ethical principle and drawing on real life scenarios. Considering the ethical principles in the context of dementia care may help us to understand why doll therapy is received well by those who believe it has a positive impact, while others may view it as a childish and demeaning practice.

Key ethical principles in healthcare

The topic of ethics is one that is extremely complex. Indeed, there are many textbooks and philosophical interpretations of ethics

---

1   This chapter is adapted from Mitchell and Templeton (2014).

that date back thousands of years. It is therefore beyond the scope of this chapter to give detailed consideration to the vast area of ethics in general, so this chapter offers readers an overview of the key ethical principles that are important in healthcare, and how these may help frame the use of doll therapy in dementia care.

In short, ethics is about the determination of right from wrong. This is based on knowledge as opposed to opinion. In the field of healthcare most people talk about bioethics, which has a strong focus on human life and health (Beauchamp and Childress 2009). Many healthcare professionals will be aware of the guiding bioethical principles that include autonomy, beneficence, fidelity, justice, non-maleficence and veracity (see Table 4.1).

Table 4.1: Ethical principles

Ethical principle	Definition
Autonomy	To respect a person's right to make choices
Beneficence	To do good
Fidelity	To be faithful to a person's cause or belief
Justice	To treat all equally
Non-maleficence	To do no harm
Veracity	To be truthful

Source: Beauchamp and Childress (2009)

Autonomy

Autonomy relates to respecting the decision-making capability of people (Johnstone 2006). In dementia care this can be complicated if the person living with dementia is deemed to lack capacity. In these cases, best practice recommendations are for advocates (usually healthcare professionals and the person's family) to make complex medical decisions based on the person's best interest. These might relate to things such as completing 'Do Not Resuscitate Orders', adapting a person's prescribed medication in light of new symptoms, or adaption of a person's environment to promote independence. While acting on the principle of best interest is important as it maintains the safety of the person living with the advancing symptoms of dementia, it should be noted that people living with dementia should never have decisions about their life and care made on their behalf as an automatic rule. People living with dementia should always be supported to engage in shared decision-making where possible, and when the disease advances, they should still be supported to make non-complex decisions, even when they are assessed to lack capacity (Mitchell and Templeton 2014). Such non-complex decisions could include what the person likes to wear, what she wants to eat, or when she chooses to engage in an activity or not.

Beneficence and non-maleficence

Beneficence is about 'doing good' and non-maleficence is about 'doing no harm'. These two concepts often go hand in hand when considering the aforementioned bioethical principles (Butts and Rich 2008). In relation to dementia care, healthcare workers and care partners should always consider the impact of what they do in relation to the person living with dementia, and if what they do is good and does not cause harm. A common example relates to the management of distress by pharmacological means. Distressed reactions, or behaviours that can indicate physical or psychological pain/stress, are/can be a common symptom of dementia diseases. As illustrated in the opening chapter, it is common for such occurrences to be managed by pharmacological means, that is, prescription of antipsychotic, anxiolytic or sedative medications. In relation to beneficence, these prescriptions may be perceived as 'doing good' because they are limiting episodes of distress that the person living with dementia is experiencing. However, some may argue that long-term medication, particularly of antipsychotics, leads to long-term problems, including the acceleration of cognitive decline. With this in mind, healthcare professionals, and indeed care partners, must decide whether the benefits (beneficence) of an action outweigh the risk of harm (non-maleficence).

Fidelity and justice

Fidelity is about respecting a person's views and/or choices, while justice is about treating a person as an equal (Beauchamp and Childress 2009). These are important ethical tenets that are central to dementia care. With regard to fidelity, healthcare professionals and other care partners are key in relation to determining life and care preferences if the person living with dementia loses her ability/capacity to make complex decisions. Thus advance care planning can be used to reflect what the person living with dementia would have wanted when she had capacity. When considering justice, healthcare professionals, care partners and society have an ethical duty to treat all people living with dementia equally, in a way that is inclusive and does not enhance the stigma associated with the disease.

Veracity

Veracity is about truth-telling. Ethical dilemmas are commonly reported in dementia care in relation to this area. In particular, questions about whether to tell someone she has a diagnosis of dementia (Mitchell *et al.* 2013a, 2013b), and the use of 'therapeutic lying' to relieve distress (Mitchell 2014b; Tuckett 2012). While this principle suggests that healthcare professionals and care partners stick strictly to the ethical principle of veracity, or truth-telling, some may argue that this approach may cause more distress, or maleficence, for those living with dementia in some circumstances.

Ethical intepretations of doll therapy

As noted in Chapter 2, the practice of doll therapy, while in its infancy, has produced favourable results for some with dementia. On the one hand, therapeutic engagement with dolls should be promoted for people with dementia based on the principle of beneficence. Beneficence in this instance refers to the healthcare professional, or care partner, taking action to promote the welfare of the person living with dementia. The concept of beneficence, related to doll therapy, can also extend to Kitwood's positive person work (1997). As noted in Chapter 3, positive interaction, or positive person work, is a means by which communication and wellbeing for people with dementia is promoted (Kitwood 1997). In addition, positive person work identifies a number of interactions that are considered to be beneficial to people with dementia, which include play, relaxation and facilitation. These concepts are all pertinent to doll therapy, and can, to some extent, provide a rationale and support for its use.

Infantilising

While there are benefits associated with doll therapy, there may be a number of challenges with regard to its use, as some may believe it to be a demeaning practice for those living with dementia and their families (Boas 1998; Salari 2002). The most common theme of contention has been identified as infantalising, that is, treating people with dementia as though they are children (Andrew 2006) or as a parent might treat their very young child (Kitwood 1997). Notably, Kitwood (1997) identified a number of depersonalising tendencies that healthcare professionals routinely exhibited, which resulted in undermining the personhood of those living with dementia. These were largely based on ignorance, as healthcare professionals did not always recognise that the person with dementia was, as Kitwood termed, an agent who could make things happen in the world. As discussed in Chapter 3, Kitwood referred to these practices as malignant social psychology, which is based on stigmatisation rather than acts of purposeful cruelty. With reference to the use of doll therapy, Kitwood identified infantilisation as behaviour worthy of being referred to in his theory of malignant social psychology.

It should be noted that many authors attribute the theoretical underpinnings of doll therapy in the work of developmental psychology (Loboprabhu *et al.* 2007; Miesen 1993) with a particular focus on the work of child psychologists (Bowlby 1967; Winnicott 1953). These theoretical underpinnings arguably add weight to the claim that the application of doll therapy may be considered child-like in nature. As stated, while there may be potential for benevolent action (beneficence) consistent with Kitwood's positive person work, there is also a risk of labelling the act as malevolent (non-maleficence), or as doing harm by means of infantilising the older person with dementia. As person-centred care seeks to move away from infantilisation of the older person, a key facet of malignant social psychology, this presents a dilemma for healthcare professionals and care partners to deliberate. The key here may lie in the fact that doll therapy is thought of as 'play' in the context of dementia care, as opposed to a creative way to communicate with someone of diminished capacity, which is how it is understood in child developmental psychology.

Autonomy

A further important area for ethical consideration is that of autonomy or choice. The ideology of person-centred care in the health arena is founded on the notion that all human beings are worthy of respect, irrespective of their disability (Butts and Rich 2008). The principle of autonomy relates to the freedom of a person to self-determine her own course of action. In other words, the person with dementia should be free to choose, and entitled to act on, her preferences, so long as these decisions and actions do not stand to violate, or impinge on, the significant moral interests of others (Beauchamp and Childress 2009). Due to the advancing disease, people living with dementia may not be able to maximise their previous level of autonomy, for example, choosing which medicines are most appropriate for their care (Mitchell *et al.* 2014). Yet, despite this cognitive decline, people living with dementia need to be supported to make non-complex decisions, for example, what to choose to eat for dinner. Doll therapy may be considered a non-complex decision for a person living with dementia to make, as engagement or non-engagement is unlikely to cause physical harm. In relation to the therapeutic use of dolls for people with dementia, the principle of autonomy would indicate that if the person wishes to engage with a doll, she should be supported to do so.

Veracity

When considering veracity, the concept of the 'therapeutic lie' is central, and its importance/prominence in the dementia care literature has increased over recent years (Schermer 2007; Tuckett 1998, 2012; Wood-Mitchell *et al.* 2008). In short, a therapeutic lie is told to someone when it is believed to be in her best interest (Culley *et al.* 2013). Like the phenomenon of doll therapy, the 'therapeutic lie' has divided opinion in healthcare. Importantly, the two overlap when considering veracity with the practice of doll therapy. Veracity is about truth-telling, a key component of Kitwood's work on positive person work. Conversely, Kitwood considered lying to people with dementia as treachery, an undesirable facet of his theory on malignant social psychology (Kitwood 1997). The increasing realism of some dolls used in empirical research has presented occasions when people with dementia consider their dolls to be real babies (Mitchell *et al.* 2014). Advocates of doll therapy do not suggest that the therapy is presented as life-like, but that if a person with dementia considers the doll to be a baby, healthcare professionals should not try to correct this notion, and as such engage in a form of therapeutic lying. Minshull (2009) supports this notion, and believes that this non-correction should be seen as, 'An avoidance of an unnecessary truth, rather than a lie' (p.36). According to Tuckett (2012), the therapeutic lie can be understood in the context of compassion and fulfilling a part of beneficence if it is in the best interests of the person with dementia, and subsequently serves to promote her wellbeing. Despite the potential for beneficence, there are many who believe that veracity is an important component of dementia care, as well as person-centred care.

Informed consent

While engaging with dolls may seem physically harmless to some, there have been indications to suggest it has the potential to divide ethical opinion (Boas 1998; Salari 2002). In this context of doll therapy and autonomy, healthcare professionals may need to think about the process of informed consent. This process is challenging when considering someone with advancing dementia. However, in spite of this challenge, it is appropriate to make an individualised care plan for engagement of this therapy as effectiveness, or engagement with this, may change over time. As alluded to, the person with dementia may lack cognitive capacity and be unable to make complex decisions about her care. In such circumstances, a family member and healthcare professional will usually act as an advocate for the person with dementia where complex decisions are necessary, for example, when to begin taking additional food supplements with meals to reduce weight loss. While doll therapy is considered harmless, it can be distressing for family to witness. As person-centred care also places an emphasis on care of the patient's relatives, it is recommended that they are involved in the decision-making process about doll therapy. In addition, in order to maintain professional conduct, it may be appropriate for healthcare professionals to gain written consent from relatives for the continual practice of doll therapy.

Fatigue

It has also been shown that over-engagement with dolls can lead to fatigue and exhaustion for the person with dementia. And severe distress can occur if the person with dementia loses her doll, or believes that her doll has died (Mitchell *et al.* 2014). There is also the potential for distress from family members who may perceive that doll therapy is undignified. As demonstrated, the concept of person-centred care can be an ambiguous term for some healthcare professionals. Despite this, there is a shared set of values that are intrinsic to the person-centred approach. These closely mirror Kitwood's work (1997) and the ideology of positive person work for people with dementia, and include getting to know the patient as a person, enabling the patient to engage in shared decision-making about treatments, therapies and lifestyle choices, and providing information that is individually tailored to each person in order to assist in decision-making and supporting the person to carry out her decisions (Mitchell and Templeton 2014). While complex decision-making may be reduced for people with advancing dementia, the selection of non-complex therapies should be encouraged and supported by healthcare professionals and care partners. While we may wish to encourage people with dementia to make their own autonomous decisions, we must also recognise that these decisions may have consequences.

So, therapeutic engagement with dolls can be beneficial to the general level of wellbeing that a person living with dementia experiences, but despite this potential for beneficence, ethical contentions around the phenomenon continue to exist. As illustrated in Chapter 2, doll therapy can assist people with dementia in communication, increase their levels of engagement with other people and reduce episodes of distress. Beneficence is arguably further reinforced when considered alongside personal autonomy. As a result, the person with dementia should be supported to make her own decision about a non-complex therapy involving dolls. While these principles of beneficence and autonomy are supported by Kitwood's positive person work and the concept of person-centred care, admittedly they do not automatically supersede non-maleficence and veracity. The perception of doll therapy as 'play' has connotations that may result in treating the person with dementia who engages with dolls like a child. This notion is contraindicated in person-centred care and Kitwood's positive person work.

The importance of advocacy then becomes a vital consideration for nursing professionals caring for a vulnerable population, people with dementia. Healthcare professionals and care partners can/ may then occupy a difficult position relating to the phenomenon of doll therapy for those with dementia. The tendency to either advocate or discourage doll therapy can therefore be supported through the ethos of person-centred care, positive person work and well-known bioethical principles.

Human rights

As argued, healthcare professionals and care partners may be faced with particular ethical dilemmas that impact on how they think about and care for people with dementia who engage with dolls. The significance of ethical decision-making around this therapeutic technique is that there are currently no right or wrong solutions, no uniform responses that must be made, merely instinctive judgements about how to act and react. Subjective ethical decision-making is an important consideration, particularly when healthcare professionals are confronted with a situation for which they are unprepared, do not understand and may lack training (Kelly and Innes 2013). Such personalised justifications are shaped and influenced by the interactions of numerous factors including personal beliefs, values, knowledge and experience (Butts and Rich 2008). Consequently, how people conceptualise and define what is 'ethical' and indeed 'unethical' varies between individuals (Beauchamp and Childress 2009). In the dementia care arena, this may result in the person with dementia being viewed and treated differently depending on a healthcare professional's personal choices, and how he personally resolves and settles his ethical dilemmas around doll therapy (Mitchell and Templeton 2014).

To conduct oneself ethically generally requires treating others with respect, doing 'good' and causing no harm, based on a personal choice to do so. Rights entitlements, on the other hand, are not based on personal choices to be applied or not, but are actual legal claims and internationally agreed standards that influence and determine the morality of the current social context. In this sense, considering dementia patients as rights holders can empower healthcare professionals to resolve their ethical dilemmas through the prospect of making tangible improvements in the lives of those with dementia. Regrettably, however, dementia patients' ability to claim and protect their rights may be compromised, exposing them to greater risk of abuse, violence, injury, neglect, maltreatment and exploitation (Freeman 2011). For this reason, changing attitudes towards people with dementia remains a fundamental responsibility and challenge for social and health care service providers.

Internationally, adoption of the World Programme for Action Concerning Disabled Persons (Division of Economic and Social Information and the Centre for Social Development and Humanitarian Affairs 1983) paved the way for a new approach to raise awareness about the need to recognise and respect the rights of people with dementia. Applying the jurisprudence of the Convention on the Rights of Persons with Disabilities (UN General Assembly 2007) has advanced the international normative framework on disability greatly. Promoting a rights-based culture within dementia care may ensure high quality and uniform services that can support a greater understanding of a controversial and potentially beneficial therapeutic technique such as doll therapy. General principles of the Convention pertinent to the phenomenon of doll therapy include, 'respect for inherent dignity, individual autonomy, including the freedom to make one's own choices, and respect for differences and acceptance of others as part of human diversity' (Article 3). Interestingly, with regards to potential interventions, as outlined in Article 4(f), state parties should:

> undertake or promote research and development of universally designed goods, services, equipment and facilities, which should require the minimum possible adaptation and the least cost to meet the specific needs of a person with disabilities, to promote their availability and use, and to promote universal design in the development of standards and guidelines…[and]…to promote the training of professionals and staff working with persons with disabilities so as to better provide the assistance and services guaranteed by those rights.

Finally, states also have an obligation to provide 'appropriate measures to ensure their freedom of expression and opinion, and access to information through all forms of communication of their choice and accepting augmentative and alternative communication, and all other accessible means' (Article 21, UN General Assembly 2007). Doll therapy may be viewed as one such low-cost, easily accessible means that not only enables dementia patients to communicate and express their views, but has also been shown to increase their wellbeing. Applying a rights-based approach can furnish healthcare professionals with an understanding, rationale and a framework on which to base their person-centred ethical decisions.

Ethical case scenarios

Thus far this chapter has shed light on the rationale behind the varied ethical interpretations on the use of doll therapy in dementia care. The application of this knowledge, as it pertains to ethical decision-making, may be more complex in practice. The following section provides some scenarios that can be used to guide healthcare professionals and care partners on decision-making in relation to doll therapy in dementia care.

Scenario 1

Ethel has lived with dementia for over five years. She currently lives in a specialist dementia care unit in a nursing home. The care staff noted how in recent weeks Ethel's level of wellbeing increased following the introduction of a doll. When visiting their mother, Ethel's two daughters, Karen and Jane, expressed concern that their mother was playing with a child's toy. They asked the care staff to remove the doll immediately. The care team complied with the family's request, removed the doll, and Ethel began to become distressed.

Analysis of scenario 1

This scenario can be common in clinical practice. Karen and Jane's interpretation of doll therapy is based on their own personal feelings, which are understandable, given the content of this chapter. Care staff have a duty of care to both Ethel and to her daughters. As such, care staff should provide tailored education to Ethel's family about the benefits of doll therapy that Ethel is experiencing, and how removal of the doll has the potential to cause distress. It is important to note that Ethel has made her own decision, a non-complex one, in relation to engagement with the doll, and should therefore not be forcibly separated from it. In future, the care staff should communicate with the care partners of residents living with dementia who are benefiting from doll therapy. That way, care partners can be assured that doll therapy not only has its place in dementia care, but can also result in a vast array of benefits for the person living with dementia.

Scenario 2

Mary has recently been admitted to hospital for a fall. She has been on the unit for a few weeks, but appears more confused recently. One of the nurses on the unit suggested that the staff try creative approaches to help alleviate Mary's distress. One of the suggested creative approaches suggested was doll therapy. When presented with the doll, Mary said that she did not want to engage with the doll. The hospital team, aware of the benefits of doll therapy, left the doll with Mary anyway because they thought it may take some time to make a positive impact.

Analysis of scenario 2

In this scenario the hospital team should be praised for considering non-pharmacological approaches for managing Mary's distress. While numerous positive outcomes have been associated with doll therapy, it is imperative to note that not all people living with dementia, or even the majority, will derive therapeutic benefit from a doll. When Mary declined to engage with the doll, care staff should note her preference and respect her decision. Importantly, this does not mean that Mary will not derive therapeutic connection with a doll in the future, but, on this occasion, the hospital staff should consider other approaches.

Scenario 3

George was diagnosed with young-onset dementia a few years ago. George currently lives in a care home and has derived therapeutic benefit from his doll, Jacob, for the past few years. Recently George has become distressed during mealtimes because he is separated from Jacob during these periods. The care home manager has forbidden the doll from being in George's presence during mealtimes because George's appetite has reduced, and his oral intake has been decreasing over the last number of months.

Analysis of scenario 3

This scenario presents a number of ethical dilemmas. On the one hand, George is losing weight, and while this is part of the expected trajectory of the dementia diseases, it is something that healthcare professionals must seek to address. Providing George with an environment that is free from distraction could enhance his level of concentration and independence at mealtimes, therefore increasing his mealtime experience and nutritional intake. Unfortunately, this is not the case for George, who is distressed because he wants to be reunited with his doll. As demonstrated in Chapter 2, doll therapy has been associated with increased nutritional intake. With this in mind, doll therapy could be trialled during George's mealtime. This is what George wants, is likely to alleviate distress, and may actually improve George's interest in food and his mealtime experience. Care staff should be advised that George might wish to 'feed' his doll, as has been reported in empirical research studies. This has the potential to work well if George 'shares' the food with his doll, that is, George has a spoonful and then provides the doll with a spoonful.

Scenario 4

Doll therapy is currently practised within a dementia care unit. There are a number of residents who believe their doll is actually a baby and call their doll by different names. Some members of the care team go along with what the residents say, and refer to the dolls by their given names, while other members do not believe they should go along with this because it feels like lying to residents.

Analysis of scenario 4

While there is much debate around 'therapeutic lying' in dementia care, the approach of 'validation' has been one that has been advocated by many dementia experts for years. In short, 'going along with what a resident says' can be interpreted as 'validation', that is, acceptance of that person's reality. As noted in Chapter 1, validation was developed by Naomi Feil (1982, 1993) as a way in which healthcare professionals, and indeed care partners, could be empathetic to people living with dementia. While telling lies is not advisable or morally right, telling the resident that her doll is a baby can be ethically justified if you are validating what the person living with dementia is already saying. To go against what the person living with dementia perceives can cause greater distress and negatively impact that resident's life, and so is never advisable.

Scenario 5

Irene has been living with dementia for over six years and is currently in supported living accommodation. Irene has a child's doll that she cuddles from time to time. One of Irene's carers questions whether or not this is right, as the evidence underpinning doll therapy is not related to children's dolls. The care worker also feels that the children's doll infantilises Irene, and could enhance the stigma of living with dementia.

Analysis of scenario 5

The care worker is correct – the dolls that are usually associated with doll therapy are anatomically accurate or empathy dolls. A child's doll (i.e. a plastic doll made by a manufacturer of children's toys) is not normally recommended. That being said, the care worker should be aware that Irene may not practice doll therapy in a conventional way, that is, the child's toy may represent a significant attachment for reasons that the care worker is unable to understand. If a bond has developed between Irene and her doll, this should not normally be broken. Should the care worker wish to encourage Irene to use an empathy or anatomically accurate doll, the care worker must offer Irene this choice (i.e. without taking the plastic doll away first). It is important to have Irene's consent throughout the entire process.

Scenario 6

Bobby has been using doll therapy for a number of years, and has experienced a number of benefits in relation to his independence and wellbeing. Over the past few months Bobby appears to have less energy as the dementia disease progresses. Bobby can become distressed when he is not with the doll because for the past few years he has rarely been detached from it. Bobby takes the doll to the bathroom, to the lounge areas and to bed. Bobby has become more distressed in recent months – he thought that the doll was a baby that had died; he was worried that the baby was not getting enough to eat because it was spitting out its food; and he worried that he would not be able to find someone to look after the baby when he got older.

Analysis of scenario 6

Bobby's holistic health is important to consider here. On the one hand, his physical health is deteriorating and he appears to becoming exhausted, caring for the doll. But removing the doll completely is likely to cause distress due to the bond between Bobby and his doll. It is likely that Bobby's holistic health would benefit in time if the doll was more therapeutic. In this scenario there is no automatic correct outcome. However, it is recommended that the care staff support Bobby in the areas where he is struggling by validating his fears and assuring him that they can care for his doll at different parts of the day, providing Bobby with an opportunity to rest and retain his therapeutic attachment with the doll.

Conclusion

While there is much controversy surrounding the practice of 'doll therapy', there is little doubt that some people with dementia benefit greatly from its use. The paucity of empirical research on its optimum use in clinical practice, coupled with inconsistent practices and lack of guidelines, has led to a limited knowledge base among healthcare professionals about the phenomenon. As demonstrated through the multiple lenses of bioethics and Kitwood's work, doll therapy can be viewed as a positive or negative engagement. Irrespective of health professionals' interpretation, they are duty-bound to keep the person with dementia at the core of the dilemma, taking into consideration Kitwood's positive person work and how it applies to the concept of autonomy, and the social/moral justice ideal of respecting and upholding the human rights of the person with dementia. Such a person-centred approach may offer a framework that supports health professionals in negotiating their personal ethical dilemmas about doll therapy as they assist people with dementia to make their own choices.

Chapter 5

Palliative Care, Dementia and Doll Therapy

Gary Mitchell and Helen Kerr

In the previous chapters doll therapy in dementia care has been considered with reference and application to bioethical principles, person-centred care and the pioneering work of the late Professor Tom Kitwood. This chapter considers the application of doll therapy to palliative care, which is, put simply, a human right for all people living with dementia. This chapter provides an overview of the concept of palliative care, illuminates ways in which palliative care is optimised for people living with dementia, and finally, how therapeutic engagement with dolls may indeed form a key part in the provision of palliative care for some people living with dementia.

Background

Globally, it is estimated that every year over 20 million people will require palliative care at the end of life. Sixty-nine per cent are adults aged over 60, highlighting that the majority of palliative care needs dominate in the older age group, with dementias, cardiovascular diseases, cancer and chronic obstructive pulmonary disease (COPD) among the conditions that carry the burden of end of life palliative care (WHO 2014). Palliative care is defined as:

> an approach that improves the quality of life of patients and their families facing the problems associated with life-threatening illnesses, through the prevention and relief of suffering by means of early identification and impeccable assessment and treatment

of pain and other problems, physical, psychosocial and spiritual. (WHO 2002, p.1)

Palliative care focuses on providing care to patients with a serious illness from which he is not expected to recover (NCPC 2006). The overarching aim of palliative care is to improve the quality of life for those with an advanced non-curative condition (DHSSPS 2010) by addressing the physical, emotional and spiritual needs (Sepulveda *et al.* 2002) in addition to their social needs (NCPC 2006).

Although managing pain and other symptoms such as fatigue, constipation and nausea are crucial, palliative care also looks at the person as a whole, using a person-centred approach, and adopts a holistic approach to care (DHSSPS 2010). In embracing a holistic approach with the patient, palliative care also aims to address the psychosocial and supportive care needs for families (WHO 2007).

One of the challenges in palliative care has been determining when it is made available, as there can be a blurring regarding when the transition between curative and palliative care takes place (DHSSPS 2010). There is increasing support for early referral for palliative care (Clarke 2002; McNamara, Rosenwax and Holman 2006; Sepulveda *et al.* 2002; WHO 2007). Early referral has been developed from a greater understanding that difficulties experienced at the end of life may have their origins at an early time in the trajectory of disease (Sepulveda *et al.* 2002); therefore, 'there is an impetus to move palliative care further upstream in the disease progression seeking integration with curative and rehabilitation therapies and shifting the focus beyond terminal care' (Clarke 2002, p.906). WHO (2007) has said that ideally palliative care services should be available from the time of diagnosis of a life-threatening illness such as cancer. An early referral, however, is dependent on the patient's need, choice and availability of resources (McNamara *et al.* 2006).

Another challenge has been expanding the focus of palliative care to other illnesses in addition to the cancer population. Although cancer is the underlying cause in 25 per cent of deaths, interestingly, 95 per cent of those who access specialist palliative care services have cancer (NCPC 2009). While the need for palliative care has been acknowledged worldwide in the cancer population from the early 1980s (WHO 2014), in recent years the need for palliative care for other chronic diseases or life-threatening conditions has been increasingly acknowledged (Murtagh *et al.* 2004; WHO 2014). In the UK, for example, palliative care has mostly been provided for people with cancer, while it is argued that those with a non-cancer diagnosis have comparable palliative care needs (Murtagh *et al.* 2004). The growing interest in extending the benefits of palliative care to those with diseases other than cancer aims to make 'palliative care for all a reality' (Clarke 2002, p.906). Although WHO (2007) states that patients with cancer in the advanced stages would generally have the greatest needs for palliative care, it is recognised that individuals with other conditions, such as dementia, and their families also need palliative care (van der Steen *et al.* 2014), with WHO (2014) encouraging countries to ensure an expansion of palliative care to patients with other life-threatening illnesses.

The modern hospice movement is widely considered to have developed from the work of Dame Cicely Saunders, with the opening of St Christopher's Hospice in London in 1967. This laid the basis for the development of modern hospice and palliative care services (Clarke 2002), with many voluntary hospices demonstrating excellence in end of life care since the foundation of the modern hospice movement (DH 2008). Hospices offer care for people facing a life-limiting illness by an interdisciplinary team and trained volunteers, providing medical care as well as emotional and spiritual support (NHPCO 2013).

End of life care is a key component of the wider concept of palliative care and, therefore, many of the same principles apply (DHSSPS 2010). It is 'described as the period of time during which an individual's condition deteriorates to the point where death is either probable or would not be an unexpected event within the ensuing 12 months' (DHSSPS 2010, p.22). While some people will benefit from palliative care at varying stages of their illness, palliative care within the last 12 months of life is regarded as end of life care (NICE 2011). Palliative care continues into end of life care as both approaches are on the same continuum (DHSSPS 2010). Physical symptoms such as pain, nausea and constipation, in addition to psychological, social and spiritual care, continue to be assessed and managed in end of life care, along with supporting families'/carers' needs. Individuals with advanced life-threatening illnesses and their families should expect good end of life care, whatever their condition (NICE 2011).

Although palliative care is a relatively new component to modern healthcare, it is being increasingly recognised as an essential part of all healthcare systems (WHO 2014). Palliative and end of life care has improved over recent years (DHSSPS 2010), but it is widely acknowledged that there is still inadequate access to hospice and palliative care worldwide (WHO 2014). Public knowledge of palliative care also remains limited (McIlfatrick *et al.* 2014), possibly in part due to palliative medicine only being introduced as a specialty in the UK in 1987 (Clarke 2014). Increasing public and professional awareness and understanding of what palliative and end of life care is, is a key component to the development of high quality care (DHSSPS 2010), although as a society, death and dying is still not talked about openly (DH 2008).

Palliative care in dementia

While hospice and palliative care programmes have often focused on the needs of people living with cancer, it is now recognised that the majority of those needing palliative care are diagnosed with non-malignant conditions (Mitchell and Twycross 2015). In relation to palliative care, three main disease types emerged – cancer, organ failure (including heart failure and COPD) and dementias (Lunney *et al.* 2003). Typically these are, first, a trajectory with a consistent steep decline (often as a result of cancer); second, a trajectory with a general decline over time but with peaks and troughs in levels of functioning (often as a result of organ decline, e.g. heart failure or COPD); and third, a trajectory with a gradual decline over a longer period of time (often as a result of advancing age and dementia). The challenges of palliative care associated with the dementia diseases are often due to the gradual decline over time, meaning that the 'terminal' or dying phase is often difficult to define. Incidentally, this is contrasted with cancer, when the terminal phase often causes a dramatic and marked reduction in the abilities and independence of the person (Mitchell *et al.* 2016).

As palliative care is different from end of life care, within the dementia care arena, its availability should be considered an option, if appropriate, from diagnosis, because it affords the person the greatest opportunity to contribute to the planning of his care before his disease progresses. The completion of an advance care plan is often advocated. This is defined as a voluntary discussion about the future care between the patient, his doctors and or nurses and the family or care partners of the patient, and it identifies the person's preference around the type of care he may or may not wish to receive, which includes preferences around his death (Harrison-Dening, Jones and Sampson 2011).

In dementia care one of the most important aspects of palliative care relates to pain management. This is because many people with dementia often have co-morbidity conditions that may cause pain, such as arthritis, pressure sores, urinary tract infections or constipation (Hughes *et al.* 2007; Mitchell 2014). It is estimated that approximately 40 per cent of older people who are cognitively impaired require pain relief, with this rising to over 80 per cent before their death (Chatterjee 2012). As communication deteriorates as part of the disease process of dementia, the person living with dementia may not be able communicate his level of pain. As a result, pain is often unrecognised and therefore not treated (Jones and Mitchell 2015). Unfortunately people living with dementia are often treated with the wrong medications (i.e. antipsychotic medications or sedative medications instead of analgesia) as they exhibit signs of distress that are associated with pain. This could manifest as distress, which could include behavioural changes, restlessness and vocalisation (Mitchell and Agnelli 2015a, 2015b). A key part of palliative care is therefore ensuring that the person living with dementia experiences as little pain as possible, so regular administration of PRN analgesia is very important, along with regular assessment.

A number of assessment tools can be used to measure and/ or assess pain in people with dementia. The gold standard is to ask the person living with dementia if he is in pain, and on a scale of 1–10, what his level of pain is. In the advance stages of the disease, where the person may no longer be articulate feelings of pain, it is best practice to use a validated pain assessment tool, such as the Abbey Pain Scale, which enables practitioners to predict the person's level of pain (Roger 2006). If the current prescription of analgesia is not effective, it is the nurse's responsibility to contact the resident's GP or specialist palliative care team for a more potent medication, a transdermal patch (which can be beneficial if the person has difficulty swallowing) or a syringe driver for use in the advance stages of the disease. Practitioners may wish to familiarise themselves with the WHO (1996) pain ladder, which is a simple guide for pain relief – namely, if pain occurs there should be a prompt administration of non-opioid medications as a first-line treatment (e.g. Aspirin or Paracetamol), then, if pain is still present, progression should be made to mild opioids as a second treatment (e.g. Codeine or Oxycodone), and if pain persists, strong opioids (e.g. Morphine or Fentanyl).

While the physical care of a person who is dying is extremely important, as noted above, there should also be a consistent focus on the psychological, social and spiritual needs of the person in fulfilling true holistic care (Mitchell 2015). Notably the ethos of holistic care corresponds directly with person-centred care theory, which is already well developed in dementia care through Tom Kitwood's work, as discussed earlier. In short, people living with dementia may become anxious, distressed or depressed throughout the remainder of their life (DH 2009, 2010). Provision of true person-centred care can be beneficial, and activities such as talking to the person, using touch, providing meaningful activity and reminiscence therapy should be embedded into care home practices (DH 2009, 2010).

Effective communication is ultimately the medium for which these best practices flourish (McGreevy 2016). Spirituality can be difficult to define and is not always related to religious beliefs, although these may be a key part of it. Wynne (2013) highlights the importance of spirituality throughout the lifespan, but particularly at the end of life, explaining that spiritual care conjoins the physical, psychological and social aspects of progressive illness;

in turn, meeting individual spirituality needs improves the ability to cope with ill health.

Palliative care and doll therapy in dementia care

It might seem puzzling to consider doll therapy in dementia care as something associated with palliative care. Indeed, palliative care, dementia and doll therapy are topics that are seldom considered together. This is hardly surprising given that the empirical evidence on palliative care, which suggests that many healthcare professionals who do not have specialist knowledge in palliative care often struggle to adequately meet the end of life needs of people living with dementia in general.

Doll therapy in dementia care has the potential to fulfil a number of elements associated with palliative care, in particular, a person's psychological and social needs, as illustrated in Chapter 2. To summarise, doll therapy has the potential to reduce episodes of distress and enhance the overall wellbeing of some living with dementia. These improvements may negate the need for pharmacological intervention for distressed reaction, anxiety or depression.

As alluded to many times throughout this chapter, the concepts of palliative care and person-centred care are synonymous in many ways, as both seek to maximise the holistic health of people. While there are differences, remember that palliative care is applicable to every single person living with dementia because the dementia diseases are progressive, incurable and life-threatening. There are accounts of people with dementia who have engaged with doll therapy passing away with their doll beside them in bed, or who have been buried with their doll, or in some cases having ownership of the doll transfer to family members after death, as a memento of the person's final years.

Conclusion

Palliative and end of life care in dementia is an important healthcare priority due to the increasing number of people who are living with the disease. Healthcare professionals must consider many elements in relation to optimising palliative care for the person living with dementia, and these include the person's biological, psychological, social and spiritual needs. These holistic needs are complimentary and all are important. With consideration to doll therapy, the empirical evidence base suggests that psychological and social needs can be met through the provision of non-pharmacological approaches such as doll therapy. In short, engaging with dolls can be a profoundly therapeutic experience for some people living with dementia. As highlighted, the positives associated with doll therapy can be applied to long-standing, advocated and ethically responsible concepts such as person-centred care and palliative care.

Chapter 6

Newcastle Doll Therapy Programme

Ruth Lee and Ian Andrew James

The people involved in the Newcastle Challenging Behaviour Team (NCBT), led by Professor Ian Andrew James, are pioneers in the field of doll therapy in dementia care, as demonstrated by their work over the last decade. As noted in Chapter 2, the team's clinical work and research around doll therapy is internationally renowned, and has paved the way for the evolution of doll therapy within dementia care. The Newcastle team's work has greatly enhanced understanding of the therapy in dementia care. This chapter, written by two prominent members of the team, provides an overview of the development of their Doll Therapy Programme over the last decade.

Background

Our interest in doll therapy began in early 2004 when a member of the Newcastle Challenging Behaviour Team (NCBT), Lorna Mackenzie, arrived back from a care home with the sad tale of the 'dead' teddy bear. This tale involved an 85-year-old woman with dementia (Mary), who, six months earlier, had been given a new teddy by her son. He was going to spend time away on the oil rigs, but before leaving he asked his mother to look after the bear while he was gone. Mary keenly accepted the role and dutifully fed, clothed and cared for the toy. Receiving so much love, the bear soon became dirty from all the forced-feeding and handling. So, periodically at night, the staff would take away the stuffed animal to wash it. However, on the last occasion when it came out of the washing machine, its stuffing had disintegrated and it was ragged and limp. When Mary saw the saggy bear the following morning, she cried out: 'My baby is disabled, it's dead!'

Lorna's involvement in this case came as a consequence of the woman's grief reaction because, as a result of the trauma, Mary stopped eating, refused to leave her room or to take medication; she had become depressed! As is typical in the NCBT's approach, Lorna used the Newcastle framework to help the care staff understand Mary's needs. The framework involves an 8–12-week intervention (James 2011), comprised of the following four phases: background assessment; assessment of triggers and behaviour; information-sharing session; and interventions.

Phase 1: Background assessment
The gathering of information relating to Mary's background from friends, family, caregivers and from case files and relevant databases. Lorna gathered the assessment material, with the assistance of Mary's key worker.

Phase 2: Assessment of triggers and behaviour
Information was obtained to determine the events or situations that were eliciting the behaviours; this was done through discussion and completion of behavioural charts. These charts also provided in-depth information regarding each 'problem' behaviour.

Phase 3: Information-sharing session (aka formulation session)
Lorna collated the information and set up a meeting with the people involved in Mary's care (including staff, family and other professionals) to develop a shared understanding of why Mary was displaying the various behaviours. Typically such sessions change the carers from being problem- to solution-focused in their thinking. This is done by increasing empathy and improving understanding of the person's behaviours.

Phase 4: Interventions
Interventions were based on the group's suggestions from the information-sharing session, then developed and refined within a care plan. Further ongoing support was then provided for four weeks (negotiated with the care home staff) to ensure appropriate implementation of the treatment strategies; tweaking of the care plans was undertaken where necessary.

During Mary's information-sharing session, one of the support workers suggested simply replacing the teddy with an identical one. Although Lorna applauded the idea, she was concerned that they could simply get involved in a cyclical problem due to the fragility of using a stuffed toy. Some staff also raised further concerns that the bear was an infection risk. Lorna then came up with the idea of substituting the teddy with a more robust hard-bodied doll, which could be washed and disinfected regularly. And so, armed with a potential solution, but somewhat concerned about the ethics of the plan, she came back to discuss the notion with the rest of the NCBT.

Fortunately, one of her team knew of a published article on the use of dolls in dementia care (Moore 2001), but none of the clinicians had ever used the intervention before. So, with the help of this article, and via the process of Newcastle framework, a 20-inch hard-bodied doll was purchased for £12 from a local toy store, and placed in Mary's room. Within hours of its introduction, Mary was holding and cuddling the toy. She engaged with the doll in the same way she had done with the teddy. Her mood lifted, her agitation decreased, and she started to eat again.

Thus far the story seems unremarkable, as it is merely the story of a good therapist working collaboratively with care home staff, and having an interesting idea about how to meet the client's need through substituting one toy with another, more robust, one. However, what is perhaps different in this case is the nature of the NCBT's response to the 'unusual' intervention, because it demonstrates a model of working specifically designed to improve clinical practice and empower therapists to develop/enhance their interventions. Indeed, from this single case, the NCBT went on to publish seven articles on the use of doll therapy, gave presentations at over twenty conferences, and published a series of guidelines on the use of dolls.

In order to explain how this case blossomed into the large research portfolio, it is necessary to describe the structure of the NCBT, because it was deliberately set up to identify and promote this type of 'practical' intervention.

Structure and process features of the NCBT

The NCBT was set up in 1999 by a psychologist and mental health nurse, and run from within a psychology service. This location provided a backdrop in which research and audits were common features of clinical practice. The timing of the formation of the team was critical because the field of dementia had just begun to accept the need to develop alternatives to medications, although it would be another ten years before there was a unified call for the reduction of antipsychotics in the UK (Banerjee 2009).

The team was originally a care home liaison service, and some of its key remits were to:

- treat challenging behaviour in a competent and carer-centred, person-focused manner

- provide a biopsychosocial model of care in which pharmacological and non-pharmacological interventions were given as part of a rational treatment plan

- treat challenging behaviours in the setting in which they are exhibited because the settings are often linked to the behaviours, working collaboratively with care facilities to improve the wellbeing of people in care

- prevent unnecessary admissions to hospital, and facilitate discharges.

The proposed service was initially met with some scepticism, and some clinicians were disconcerted about the high level of input the team was proposing to provide to each client. The team's response to this point was that if this was any other client group, particularly a child or someone with a learning disability, the level of input they were proposing would be perceived as low.

Owing to the success of the service, and its successful role in reducing hospital admissions, the NCBT grew in size. From the outset, however, it was concerned about the degree of stress involved in working exclusively in care homes – clinician burnout being a potential risk. To prevent this, structural features were agreed with NHS management about how to run the service. For example, team members would have a relatively small caseload (n=10–12). The staff would also be provided with frequent clinical supervision (minimum of one hour a week), and they would operate within a separate specialist team from a single centre. The latter allowed for support and permitted informal supervision 'as and when' required. While the clinical work was to be the core task of the team, the therapists were all expected to partake in non-clinical activities. These extra activities are outlined in Figure 6.1, and involve teaching, consultancy and research.

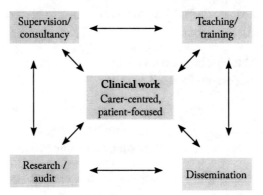

Figure 6.1: NCBT team members' activities

Teaching and consultancy were seen as essential elements of the clinical work (i.e. teaching care staff around specific cases; providing advice to psychiatrists, etc.). An important part of such roles was therapists keeping themselves up to date with new developments in the area. This married well with the research element of the team, because this was also viewed as an important feature of the NCBT's work, with each member of staff being expected to take responsibility for developing a specific area of clinical practice.

By adopting this system, the clinical team were able to publish and develop expertise in a wider range of areas, including sexuality in dementia, toileting practices, religion, aromatherapy, cognitive simulation therapy and the use of therapeutic lies. Within this research programme, doll therapy became a key area of interest for Lorna.

The research work was assisted greatly by links made to the clinical psychology course at the Universities of Newcastle and Teesside. Indeed, many of the NCBT clinicians worked with psychology trainees to produce collaborative reviews and studies.

The doll studies

Our first systematic investigation examined the use of dolls in two care homes in the North East of England. In this study, Mackenzie *et al.* (2006) found that 69 per cent of care staff reported an improvement in residents' wellbeing after the introduction of dolls. They noted improvements in resident interactions with staff, interactions with other residents, level of activity, happiness/contentment, amenability to care interventions and agitation. However, the individual profiles varied greatly, and the care staff also reported some problems using the dolls, such as disputes over ownership and dolls being mislaid.

Another descriptive study by James, Mackenzie and Mukaetova-Ladinska (2006) examined the use of dolls over a 12-week period by asking care staff to monitor doll users' levels of activity, interaction with staff and other residents, happiness and agitation following the introduction of dolls. It was found that the majority of residents who chose to use a doll obtained some benefits on these domains, but a small number of older adults appeared to obtain little, if any, beneficial effects. It was also discovered that care staff found it difficult to predict who would choose to use a doll, and 93 per cent of residents chose to use a doll in preference to a teddy bear.

A retrospective study by Ellingford *et al.* (2007) looked at the case notes of residents living in four nursing homes three months before and after the introduction of dolls by auditing residents' positive and negative behaviour recorded by staff in their daily communication records. It was found that after the introduction of dolls, doll users showed an increase in positive behaviour and a decrease in negative behaviour and incidents of aggression compared with before the dolls were introduced.

In the fourth study, Fraser and James (2008) aimed to develop an understanding of why doll therapy improves the wellbeing of older adults with dementia by interviewing eight professionals from a range of professions and residential care settings. The results suggest that the impact of the doll is grounded in complex interactions between the resident and the doll, and the residents and the wider systemic processes. A central category emerged, portraying that dolls may meet a range of basic 'individual needs' including attachment, comfort, activity, inclusion, communication/interaction, identity, innate drives, memory and fantasy. More specifically, the study results suggest that the doll may act as an attachment figure, providing direct closeness and contact, and that it provides meaningful and achievable activities by promoting the development of identity, evoking past memories of roles. It may also facilitate communication and interaction with others, encouraging inclusion. Therefore, the doll may offer an opportunity for the older adult to deal with ongoing inner psychological distress in a more adaptive way.

Despite the increasing evidence from clinical work highlighting the effectiveness of doll therapy, up to this time our work had focused solely on the professional, care staff and family caregiver perspectives rather than that of people with dementia. In response to this, in the next study (Alander *et al.* 2013), we used a grounded theory approach to conduct a series of interviews with people living in 24-hour care settings, where dolls were being used routinely. Alander interviewed sixteen participants about their views on 'the use of dolls' in two phases; five participants took part in a focus group and eleven were interviewed individually. Eight of the eleven participants had dementia, and four were actively using dolls. An analysis of their responses showed that residents supported the use of dolls, believing that they can have a positive impact on users. There were some ethical concerns raised, however, and these are discussed below.

Ethics

The main ethical issues raised in our studies related to age-appropriateness of doll use among older adults (i.e. fears of infantilisation) and potential deception where the older person believes the doll to be a real baby rather than a doll. The degree to which participants felt that doll use was an ethical intervention varied on a continuum. This highlights the complexity and confusion about the appropriateness of doll therapy. Some doll users in the Alander study were aware that the dolls were dolls, but still valued them for comfort and pleasure.

Underlying these ethical dilemmas are concerns about whether older adults' dignity is preserved. Dolls should never be forced on individuals, and not everyone will want to use them. However, allowing the person with dementia a choice about whether she would like to use a doll can be empowering. If agitation is reduced as a result of using a doll, dignity would be enhanced, rather than diminished. It could also be seen as a more preferable method than physical restraint and problematic medication.

At the heart of the ethical dilemma is how other people view and respond to doll therapy. It has long been established that the caregiver's attitude regarding treatment approaches influences therapeutic outcomes (e.g. Kitwood 1997). For example, a common concern relates to the potential misuse of dolls by 'busy' care staff, with the dolls being used to compensate for lack of human contact and comfort. Our studies have suggested that dolls' success is, in part, due to the fact that they facilitate social interaction with others. Hence, the dolls should not be treated as stand-alone devices, but rather, staff should be trained in how to make best use of them as vehicles of social engagement. Therefore, it is important that all care staff are educated about doll therapy, and given an opportunity to carefully examine their own attitudes and views related to the use of dolls in care homes.

Clinical input

From a clinical perspective we have introduced dolls into a number of care settings and have produced guidelines for the intervention based on clinical observations (Mackenzie,

Wood-Mitchell and James 2007). The introduction of doll therapy into the care homes has followed a standard format, and all care home staff receive psycho-educational training before the introduction of dolls to a home. These sessions include information about the potential psychological benefits of using dolls, behavioural and environmental strategies for minimising problems, and de-escalation techniques when problems arise.

Conclusion

The aim of this chapter has been two-fold: first, to describe some of the studies undertaken by the NCBT, the group that kick-started research into this area in a programmatic manner; and second, to demonstrate how a successful scientist-practitioner approach was established in a busy NHS clinical team. It is also worth noting that these endeavours have all been undertaken without any cost and embedded within clinical practice. It is important to highlight the symbiotic relationship between nursing and psychology, with the respective clinical and research strengths being harnessed in the production of publishable research.

Chapter 7

A Family Experience of Doll Therapy

Jessie McGreevy

This chapter provides a thoughtful account of a family's experience in relation to using doll therapy in dementia care. Jessie, a clinical support manager at Care Circle, provides a unique take on doll therapy as she reflects on how she felt as a family member some years ago. She also draws on her current specialist knowledge of dementia care, which she has gained through her clinical role today, to provide a balanced account of her opinions on doll therapy within dementia care.

Background

When someone brings up the topic of empathy dolls with me today, I know exactly what to say. I understand the benefits of using them, and I understand that it is a recognised and often successful approach to reducing distress. Additionally, I also understand that they remain a controversial therapy. With the knowledge and understanding I now have, as a nurse with 12 years' experience working in dementia settings, I have become an advocate for the use of empathy dolls for individual residents living with dementia. But this has not always been the case.

My family has been affected by dementia on several occasions throughout my lifetime. My granny was diagnosed with dementia at the ripe old age of 80, and my uncle was relatively young, at 55. Both have now passed away and had very different experiences with dementia, and both spent their last years in care homes. This year my family was affected once again by dementia, as another uncle was also diagnosed with Alzheimer's. He continues to live an independent and fulfilling life at home, and I am sure it will again be a different journey from that of his brother.

Being a dementia specialist gives me an insight into what may happen in the future, and it means the surrounding family will be equipped with better knowledge so as to ensure we can help my uncle live well for as long as possible. My professional experience has highlighted that ensuring families have knowledge is vital, especially when it comes to dementia. Dementia is a complicated illness with some of the interventions used being a bit 'outside the box' – the use of empathy dolls perhaps being one of the most difficult to understand – and understandably this can cause a lot of concern for families. As it relates to doll therapy, this was definitely the case with my family. I am delighted to have an opportunity to share my family's experience with my granny, Winnie, and her doll, 'John'.

Winnie and 'John'

Winnie was a formidable lady, had a big heart, liked things done a certain way, and was brought up in a very small village in County Down in Northern Ireland, spending all her childhood and most of her adult life on the family's farm. She married in her early twenties and had six children: three girls and three boys. Winnie always talked about how busy the house was, but she loved being a housewife, bringing up the kids, maintaining her home, baking (she made the best pancakes and Swiss rolls!) and when needed, she would roll up her sleeves and muck in on the farm.

As her children grew up, got married, left home and had kids of their own, she adopted the role of 'granny' with ease, and as she had 20 grandchildren, she was never without a child in the house. Granny was a great cook and baker; she loved having everyone over on Sundays, making sure everyone was 'fed and watered', and always sending us home with treats for school or work that week. As my granny and grandfather got older, their health started to deteriorate, and they eventually had to move out of their farm into a bungalow, which would become the new family hub.

Unfortunately, when granny was in her mid-70s, she developed some problems with her spine, and eventually had to go for corrective surgery – this is when things really changed for the family. Unfortunately the operation wasn't successful, and granny was left unable to walk independently, instead having to use a wheelchair. Shortly after this, my granny began to develop symptoms of dementia (forgetting names, becoming more withdrawn and struggling with words).

I can't remember when or how long it took for granny to get her diagnosis of dementia, but for us, as a family, things didn't really change that much after diagnosis, as we already knew what it was. This experience was almost ten years ago, so my knowledge of dementia was limited, as was the rest of the family's. Like most people in these circumstances, we were reliant on the advice of the professionals. Granny was able to live at home for a few years, but as my grandfather was getting older, the family were getting busier, and granny's symptoms were progressing, a decision was made that it would be best if she moved into a nursing home. It was a difficult decision at the time, especially for my grandfather, but looking back, it was right for both of them, as granny got the care she needed and my grandfather got a renewed sense of purpose because he enjoyed visiting the home and chatting to staff. Most importantly, my grandfather took great comfort from seeing that my granny was well cared for.

The care home granny lived in was a small private nursing home in the village that she grew up in, which was actually a real benefit for granny as she knew a lot of the care staff (most of whom were local people). In addition, the care staff already knew my granny, and they would always be reminiscing about the people they knew, sharing stories past and present. Despite the familiarity, the move into the home was not an easy one; like many people, granny found it difficult to adjust at the beginning, and even blamed the family on occasion.

Luckily, after a week or so, granny started to relish the care home environment, giving people orders, listening out for the gossip, and she loved the constant stream of family visitors bringing her her favourite chocolate bar, mint aero. Granny was happy in the care home for several years, but as her dementia progressed, she became more distressed at simple things – for example, if she forgot a word she would tell herself off, or if she didn't recognise a visitor (which became a daily problem) she would become very anxious and upset. We also began to notice that granny was becoming increasingly quiet, and when family would visit, she would ignore them or simply ask us to leave, which was not the granny we all knew. The family found this difficult to accept or understand.

When these changes began to happen we were very concerned, and I remember my aunt organising a meeting with the lead nurse of the care home to see if anything could be done, or if they perhaps knew why my granny had changed so much. As mentioned earlier, no one in the family really knew much about dementia, so we really relied on the staff. Unfortunately the care staff that looked after my granny also appeared to know little about the illness. The recurrent communication we received was mostly that these changes were normal with the illness.

During the meeting that was held with the nurse, my aunt was told that granny had been started on antipsychotic medication as she had started to refuse personal care and was becoming more unsettled. She explained that this was often the first-line treatment for treating distress, but could make people sleep more because of its side-effects. Of course at the time we just accepted what the nurse had said; after all, she was the professional. However, looking back with the knowledge I now have, I realise that in fact, this should have been the final solution, as the side-effects of antipsychotic medication can be very detrimental to people living with dementia.

As time went on, my granny's moods became very unpredictable, and she became increasingly quiet and withdrawn. Family visits at times had become very distressing, as she would shout when the family were visiting. She would ask to see her children, unaware that they were indeed present and visiting her. These elements made it particularly hard as she had now got to the point where she no longer recognised her children when they visited. I remember asking a carer one day why granny didn't know who I was, and she replied, saying, 'Her mind is disappearing.' This was not the scientific explanation I had been hoping for, and of course the response made me very scared for the future. I just kept thinking:

does that mean my granny is going to disappear altogether? I only wish that the care staff had said something more helpful such as, 'Don't worry if she doesn't know your name or exactly who you are. Just look at her smile, look at the way she holds your hand, she knows she loves you.' Such an explanation would have helped me to understand and encouraged me to visit more often.

It was around this time that the use of a doll was accidentally stumbled upon. As I said, granny began to ask for her children quite a bit, even when they were actually visiting, and she became very distressed when no one could provide her with an answer that she could accept. The carers and nurses told us that when she asked for her kids to say 'they were at school' or 'out playing'. As a family we were not comfortable lying to my granny, but the care staff explained that if we kept arguing with her, we would 'make her worse', which is not something we wanted to do.

There was one day when my aunt and I went to visit granny and we found her in her room with a china doll, rocking back and forward, cradling the doll and singing it a lullaby. On seeing this, my aunt became a little upset and even challenged the nurse on duty, asking, 'Why is Winnie playing with a doll?' The response was quite simple, 'She wanted to.' At the time I was surprised that the nurse didn't seem too phased or bothered by it, while my aunt and I both felt that it shouldn't have been allowed. We also felt that the care staff should not be encouraging people in their 90s to play with dolls. We acted on these feelings and took the doll from her, without thought. We subsequently asked that she not be given the doll again. Granny started to cry a little when the doll was taken away, but within a few minutes, was sitting eating chocolate and not concerned about the doll, so we thought that the incident was over and done with. However, that was not the case; later on that evening, another one of my aunts went to visit and found the same doll in bed beside granny. Her feelings mirrored ours – she didn't understand it, and felt the doll was inappropriate. Like us, she took the doll out of granny's bed and out of her room. The family requested to meet with the manager the next day to complain about staff treating granny 'like a child'.

The next day we attended a meeting (myself, my dad and my aunt) with the manager. We were curious to learn about who kept giving granny the doll. The manager explained how this 'doll therapy' came about. Once the manager told us about the benefits to our granny, we stopped arguing and realised that granny didn't see the doll as a toy, but rather as a source of comfort and love. The manager explained that granny was quite distressed at times, and although she had been given medication for her distress, it didn't seem to be making any difference – but the doll did.

The way in which 'doll therapy' came about was in actual fact quite accidental. My granny had been helping the care staff do some dusting, and one of the things she was given to dust was the china doll. When granny was given the doll she didn't dust it, but instead cradled it in her arms, began singing to it, stroking its face and appeared much happier than she had been for a very long time. When it was time to put the ornaments and the doll away, granny became very upset and didn't want to give it back, so the member of staff let her keep it. That day she was very proud and showed everyone the doll. It became clear that she no longer saw it as a doll but as her own child, John (the name of her eldest son).

The nurse also explained that the doll even helped granny's mealtime experiences and subsequently enabled her to eat more of her meals. The manager explained that while she didn't really understand the theory behind it, as many still don't, she was sure that granny was less distressed and more content with the doll. In short, the care staff were reluctant to remove the doll from her. Once we had the conversation, the manager even invited us to sit and watch what happened when granny was given the doll. She was right! Granny instantly came to life: she was smiling, looked more relaxed and was busy showing of her baby to everyone in the room. Initially it was difficult to get our heads around the idea of a doll being a therapy, but when we saw it in action, we couldn't argue.

Getting the rest of the family to accept and understand the doll wasn't easy; while the boys in the family seemed to accept it much quicker (especially my grandfather, who could see that it made my granny smile – that was enough evidence for him), perhaps surprisingly, the women took a lot more persuasion. It was frustrating that there was minimal information on doll therapy in dementia, and no one in the care home really understood the theory behind why it worked. Quite honestly, the only thing that persuaded family members to accept the doll was seeing it in action. After a while, the doll, or 'John', just became a normal part of everyday life. My granny would wash it, sing to it and put it to bed. It gave her back the sparkle she had lost for a while.

If granny didn't have John, perhaps because he was being washed (she would often feed the doll chocolate so it needed to be washed quite often), she would become worried and sometimes think that John had died or been kidnapped. To combat this we purchased a second identical doll to prevent this from happening. Even when my granny was dying, we made sure she had John with her. It would have been easy to take him away at this point, because she wasn't really aware of what was going on, but he had become a part of her, and we knew how much comfort she got from him. The doll lay in the bed beside her throughout the day and night. You would often see her holding tightly on to his hand; it seemed so natural for her.

As I explained at the beginning of this chapter, I had little knowledge about dementia at the time and certainly no knowledge of doll therapy. Of course now it all makes perfect sense to me. As granny's dementia was progressing, she was likely regressing back in her life and memories, and in her life there were always children. She was always busy cleaning, baking, taking us from A to B, and the move into the nursing home took that sense of purpose away from her. Those important attachments were gone, the comfort and love that she was so used to hadn't gone away, but it had changed. It was probable that granny felt abandoned at times. The doll was a substitute. It gave her all those things – responsibility, purpose, love, attachment and comfort. I believe that she felt like she belonged and was important once again.

Today, I use my personal experience with doll therapy to inform my practice. I truly empathise with people who live with dementia, and will try almost anything to enhance the wellbeing of that person. I appreciate doll therapy can be controversial and upsetting for some. When communicating about doll therapy with family, or care partners, the four key points I would give healthcare professionals are as follows:

- Pre-warn families that their loved one is using a doll, so they aren't shocked or surprised when they come to visit and see it being used. This will also allow them time to accept it and even source evidence themselves to figure out what doll therapy is, and why it is being used.

- Learn the theory behind the use of dolls in dementia care, and pass this knowledge on to family members in a clear and understandable manner. In short, doll therapy can increase the wellbeing of people living with dementia.

- Explain to the family that, in dementia care, a person's reality can be very different to what others experience, and the answer is usually to step into that person's reality rather than bringing him into the 'true reality', which can be very distressing. In other words, if the person living with dementia believes the doll is his baby, then that is what you as a family member should go along with.

- Finally, keep talking with everyone involved. It is good relationships between the person, their family and care professionals that enable people with dementia to live well. Remember that dementia affects everyone in the family – not just the person with dementia.

Chapter 8

Tales from Care

Marsha Tuffin

In this chapter, Marsha Tuffin, Head of Care and Dementia Services at Abbeyfield & Wesley (Northern Ireland), describes her own personal experiences of doll therapy within dementia care from her professional point of view.

Background

After 19 years of working for Abbeyfield in various direct care settings for older people, I can honestly say that doll therapy never ceases to amaze me. From my direct observational experiences, doll therapy has provided many benefits for some individuals living with a dementia. The therapy may, of course, still be regarded as controversial, and has at times caused distress for family members, staff and other residents due to them believing that this practice was undignified, demoralising and demeaning. However, in many instances I have witnessed improved social interactions and improvements in the overall wellbeing of people living with a dementia who engage with dolls.

Discovering doll therapy

I learned about doll therapy through studying for my degree, but personally felt, at that stage of my career, that it was a slightly patronising theory, and I also didn't truly understand how effective it could be in the real world. I mainly steered towards using animals and pets as therapy, because they were real and warm to touch. They also fulfilled the same nurturing or attachment theory associated with doll therapy.

It wasn't until an old Silver Cross pram was donated to my care home, for our reminiscence area, that I discovered how powerful doll therapy could be for some individuals living with dementia. Not really thinking about doll therapy, and seeking to fill a large space inside the pram, I bought a cheap plastic doll. I remember unwrapping the doll from its packaging and then casually walking down the corridor to put it in the pram. Without really thinking about it, I carried the doll upside down, swinging it by its leg as I walked to the reminiscence area. As I was walking, one of my residents came running towards me in an anxious state, her arms stretched wide out in front of her, clearly exhibiting concern about the hanging doll.

This lady's overall wellbeing improved massively with the introduction of the doll, and I would never have thought it could be so beneficial. She had been diagnosed with Alzheimer's disease and would usually be in distress in the afternoons as she searched for her children. At the time, all these years ago, the carers would use all the training and skills they'd learned to try and enter this lady's reality to try validate her feelings and alleviate any distress she was feeling. Sadly, we often failed, and consequently pharmacological interventions were introduced in order to reduce her anxiety.

However, we turned a corner with the arrival of the doll, and her wellbeing improved straight away. She would be seen cuddling, patting the doll's back, rocking and humming with the doll, with lots of signs of affection. Her communication improved, her speech was much calmer, she appeared much less distressed and her overall anxiety levels decreased, especially late in the afternoon. This was a massive leap forward, and over time, the medications used to treat her anxiety were even reduced and stopped.

Within such a short space of time, we learned some very important lessons. It was important to be careful how we handled a doll because, through the eyes of the person living with dementia, it was often real to her. My first experience of doll therapy was overwhelming, with many great benefits towards meeting a person's emotional and physical needs, although it did shock and dismay some residents, staff, visitors and families.

That first experience was ten years ago, and doll therapy is now widely used within Palmerston, the care home I am directly managing. The nurturing instinct is so strong and is a big part of the reason that doll therapy is so effective. However, it is important to note that doll therapy can lead to problems. Some residents grow attached to the dolls, and it has led to a few arguments between residents over ownership. Anxiety can arise if a resident cannot find a doll that has temporarily been mislaid. To combat this, we purchased extra dolls as many residents believed in the dolls and sought them out independently. Extra prams were also brought in as many wanted to touch, push and care for 'their babies' (the doll in a pram).

Very quickly we all learned that as residents would often fluctuate in and out of reality recognition, the doll should not be given directly to the person with a dementia – one minute it might be her baby, and the next it was a doll. In other words, it was up to the person living with dementia if or when she wanted to engage with the doll. Staff are trained to leave the dolls somewhere sitting in a chair where someone can easily find them when walking. I am proud to say that the carers at Palmerston empower and promote choice to our residents. If the residents want to provide care for the doll, that is okay; if not, that's also fine. The residents must not feel that they are being given too much responsibility to care for the doll, because this could cause anxiety or result in the doll being rejected.

Education about doll therapy is extremely important because, for doll therapy to work effectively, all care staff and family members need to be invested in the therapy. Staff and family members were introduced slowly to this type of therapy through training and meetings with relatives, as well as displaying literature on staff and relatives' notice boards. Support sessions were set up for families, and doll therapy was often discussed.

From my experience over the last ten years, the dolls don't need to be expensive. Normal average-priced dolls and even teddy bears can have the same impact, because it is about fulfilling attachment needs. One of the most important benefits of doll therapy, which I've seen, is providing residents with an identity and a role within their own private world, as it has allowed them the chance to care for someone again, instead of just being the person being cared for. Many residents are calmed by the dolls, and it can often create a distraction from upsetting events.

After the introduction of dolls, residents showed an increase in positive behaviour and a decrease in negative behaviour. Incidents of aggression, compared with before the dolls were introduced, were totally reduced. So the dolls were effective in reducing the negative and challenging behaviours and promoting more positive behaviours and moods.

To help me capture the actual introduction of doll therapy, a questionnaire was sent out, to the night staff in particular, to capture their main concerns and what was going on with the residents, especially late in the evening. Two months after the dolls were introduced, the questionnaire was sent back out. Staff reported benefits including a calming overall effect, a reduction in heavy pacing, increased communication and improved speech. Many of the staff expressed an opinion that the effect was the result of residents having a sense of purpose or focus given by the dolls.

A case study of positive, meaningful and dignified moments

To further illustrate the positive experiences of doll therapy in my practice, I have chosen to recount the following case study. Many people who know a bit about doll therapy may perceive it to be therapy that is only applicable to women. As demonstrated in this case study, it has the potential to be an extremely powerful therapy for men as well.

Previously, a male resident living with a dementia in his late 90s walked up and down all the corridors at Palmerston. Despite the environment being full of interesting objects for him to pick up, move around and touch, his movement/walking was constant. It was as if he was still looking or searching for something that was missing. As his speech was impaired, it was difficult for staff to understand just what he was expressing, although it was evident at times, by his body language and his facial expressions, that he was not in a state of wellbeing very often.

With his slender build and because he walked so much, it was hard to maintain his weight because he was burning more calories than he was consuming, and he was also prone to falls. In the afternoons this gentleman would walk more – often making it hard for carers or for himself to become settled at night. He was too frail for pharmacological interventions to be introduced, so we just had to look harder, observe and try to understand the world through his eyes.

When the dolls and prams were introduced to the unit I witnessed, through Dementia Care Mapping™ (DCM), a validated observational tool developed by the University of Bradford in the UK, some truly magical moments with this gentleman and the dolls. Within such moments the dolls gave him a role, identity and purpose throughout the day – he was no longer walking, searching up and down the corridors, or constantly going into other residents' bedrooms. In these moments he was nurturing and caring, his face full of achievement and satisfaction. True attachment had grown between him and the dolls. I now fully understood this man's words because he was so contented by doll therapy.

On another occasion I observed, through DCM, this gentleman to be wriggling the toes of the dolls in the pram (in order) – with his communication being so impaired, I could only make out the word 'piggy', although his actions and body language gave me goose bumps. The gentleman, previously in a state of sustained illbeing, was now able to sing the nursery rhyme 'Three little pigs went to market' to his doll. After the nursery rhyme, he even carefully covered up the dolls with, not only a blanket, but also bathing towels from his bedroom. He sought to ensure that the dolls were comfortable, safe and warm – and hidden underneath the blankets were biscuits and an unpeeled banana. These are truly magical moments that will stay with me for a very long time.

This gentleman's daughter noticed a massive improvement within her father's overall wellbeing when the dolls were first introduced. She felt that her father expressed himself through the dolls, and during her visits she found him calmer, kinder and gentler, in essence, more like his former self. Previously on visits the daughter would often find her father just pacing up and down the corridors and at times quite anxious. Since the dolls were introduced, she would often find her father nurturing a doll while sitting in an armchair, looking peaceful and contented. On occasions she would discover the doll, carefully placed in her father's bed, covered over by his duvet.

In addition to these benefits, this gentleman's weight has increased and has remained stable. This is due to him walking less and enjoying his dining experiences with the doll. Improvements have also been noted in his communication, as evidently he is less anxious when engaging with the dolls, and he also has a reduced risk of falls. This gentleman lives well with his dementia at Palmerston through doll therapy and other non-pharmacological interventions within the home's environment.

Conclusion

Doll therapy might not be right for everyone living with dementia at Palmerston, but we understand that every resident living will experience this differently, in their own unique way. By taking the time to listen and to see through the eyes of each of our residents, while also understanding their personhood, pharmacological interventions are seldom required in the first instance. As professionals we need to understand the nurturing, emotional and attachment needs of people living with dementia. We should not make assumptions from our own perspective about what is or is not appropriate, especially with using dolls as therapy. In turn, this will enable us to educate and support frontline workers and families of the benefits of using dolls, which can be amazing. Recounting my opening comment, 'doll therapy never ceases to amaze me', I can honestly say that after all these years, I'm still moved by the holistic benefits associated with the therapy, and the impact that dolls can have on some people living with dementia.

Chapter 9

Experiences of Doll Therapy

Caroline Baker

In this penultimate chapter, Caroline Baker, Director of Dementia Care at Barchester Healthcare, provides her opinions on doll therapy in dementia care.

A professional's change of mind

It was way back in 1997 when I first read an article on the use of dolls in dementia care, and my initial reaction was one of shock and distaste! Having recently attended a Dementia Care Mapping™ (DCM™) course, my immediate response was that the use of dolls in dementia care would be deeply infantilising, and so I promptly put the article in the bin without a second thought. However, only a year later, as a care home manager of a 50-bed care home, I announced a competition to decorate each of the four units with a Christmas theme. The administrator and I would decorate the reception area, which we turned into a park by bringing in a Christmas tree, a scattering of leaves (and accompanying spray frost), a sledge and a park bench. As I strolled through town to withdraw the care home's petty cash from the bank, I passed the window of Mothercare, and there, in the window, were lovely child-size squashy dolls that I purchased to sit on my sledge in their woolly hats and winter outfits! Mothercare were brilliant and loaned me two dolls until after Christmas. The dolls accompanied me back to the care home and sat on the Christmas sledge…but not for long.

So many residents engaged with the dolls and took hold of them. I would sit on the bench and chat with residents, not only about children, but also about relatives that the resident missed.

These meaningful moments took place as the residents tweaked the little noses and stroked the outfits of the dolls. They also liked to reposition the dolls' hats and make sure their trousers were smoothed straight.

It was one gentleman in particular, however, who changed my attitude to using dolls in dementia care completely. Harry[1] had only been in the home for about three months, and despite several attempts, would not verbally communicate with us at all. Harry came into the reception area and reached down for a doll, taking it into his arms before sitting quietly on the bench. As I sat by him, Harry began to not only cuddle the doll, but talked about his late wife who he missed dearly. No further words were needed at that time as we hugged each other and Harry cried in my arms.

The doll was definitely the catalyst for the outpouring of Harry's loss, and although he did not have children, the comfort he gained from the doll seemed to provide the security he needed to share his emotions with us. I was a true convert and began to introduce empathy dolls into the care homes wherever I worked. Like me, some staff initially had real reservations about introducing dolls, but quickly changed their minds when they saw how some of the residents would respond to them.

There are two further residents who will always stay in my mind, and who to this day continue to bring a smile to my face. Joe, who I had been observing as part of a DCM™ observation in a care home in Northern Ireland, seemed to become quite anxious and distressed following dinner. He was sat in a comfortable chair, but began repeatedly banging the arm of the chair with a worried look on his face. Staff passing stopped to speak to Joe and asked if they should fetch 'Bill'. At this point Joe nodded his head and I waited in anticipation to meet Bill. It transpired that Bill, along with a cuddly blanket, was a large empathy doll that Joe immediately took into his arms, wrapped the blanket around him and held him to his chest, stroking his back. His anxiety subsided immediately, and he spent the next couple of hours relaxed and happy.

---

1   All names in this chapter have been changed to protect the confidentiality of the residents.

Another lady, Annie, who I observed in a care home in Newcastle had four children. Annie gathered up all of the empathy dolls that were placed around the lounge (four in all), carrying two in each arm, cooing and talking to them as if they were her own children. As she sat in her chair, surrounded by the dolls, she stroked their hair, tweaked their noses, rubbed their feet and just beamed as she carried out her adornment of the dolls. When a cup of tea and biscuits were brought along for Annie, she shared them with her dolls, and her level of wellbeing was clear for all to see.

A few years ago, I had to take my nan to hospital (who did not have a diagnosis of dementia). She was really anxious as she sat in the front of my car, wondering what would happen and what was wrong with her. I had one of the dolls in the back seat of my car at the time, and asked if she would like to hold it while we travelled the 30-minute journey to hospital. Nan sat stroking the doll's hair and patting its bottom as we hurtled down the dual carriageway. Interestingly, the doll provided my nan with great comfort – so much so that the doll went into hospital with her!

Of course the use of dolls in dementia care is not for everyone living with dementia. As with everything else in dementia care, it is very much the choice of the individual, but I have had the pleasure of seeing exceptional results, on numerous occasions, which have helped residents who were experiencing distress and anxiety to feel a sense of security and comfort while engaging with dolls.

With dementia practice constantly evolving, there is encouraging evidence to support the use of robotic animals within dementia care. At the moment, I have similar reservations as I did with doll therapy, about how a robot seal can provide benefits to people who live with dementia. The intervention is currently being trialled, but I am not sure how many people will benefit because it is surely not a common occurrence for people to have seals in their own homes! Despite these reservations, I am sure that again, if I see it benefiting people in practice, my mind will be changed.

Chapter 10

Best Practice Guidelines

Gary Mitchell

This final chapter provides a summary of the best practice guidelines associated with doll therapy in dementia care. It provides a template of how doll therapy should be used in practice through a draft policy statement, best practice guidelines based on the empirical evidence base, and a personalised care plan. In addition, a short educational training framework for education and practice, as it pertains to doll therapy in dementia care, is also included. These elements should provide care providers with a methodology for introducing doll therapy within any context or healthcare setting.

Brief policy statement

There is a growing evidence base that supports the therapeutic use of dolls for some people living with dementia. This suggests that therapeutic engagement with doll can enhance wellbeing, reduce episodes of distress and stimulate increased communication and social interactions.

This policy affirms that all people living with dementia in our care the right to engage with dolls, or soft toys, because they may enhance that person's wellbeing. This policy informs healthcare staff of all grades, as well as family members and care partners, about how doll therapy is best implemented while providing respect for a person's privacy and dignity. All care providers who adopt this policy should provide their care staff with training and education in the appropriate use of dolls based on the contents of this book.

Supporting policy information

- Doll therapy can assist in the fulfilment of a number of psychological needs for people living with dementia, for example, attachment, comfort, inclusion, occupation, identity and love (Kitwood 1997).

- It is likely that doll therapy has its theoretical roots in Bowlby's theory of attachment (1969), Winnicott's theory on transitional objects (1953) and Miesen's application of these to people living with dementia (1993).

- Doll therapy can give people a sense of purpose, making an individual feel connected with others, and even providing her with a functioning role.

- Doll therapy can illicit profound feelings of maternal and paternal satisfaction, and has been therapeutic for both women and men.

- People living with dementia may experience difficulties in communicating their needs or emotions. There is evidence to suggest that doll therapy can aid people living with dementia to express their own feelings, for example, telling the doll how she feels, or reporting that the doll is hungry or tired, which may mirror her own feelings.

Guidelines for using doll therapy

- Inform family and healthcare professionals in the unit before introducing the dolls. Family members should be provided with a summary of the potential benefits. All parties should be made aware that when a doll is introduced and accepted by a person with dementia, it will not usually be removed.

- Family members or care partners may have concerns about doll therapy because of the perception that it is infantilising. It is often helpful to discuss these concerns with the family before beginning doll therapy.

- Care staff may also not be familiar with the practice of doll therapy in dementia care, and all should receive training or education on its use.

- It is advisable to have information about doll therapy, for example, an educational resource or a poster illustrating that the unit practises doll therapy, so that visitors to the unit are aware of the practice before entering.

- Seek to provide different styles of doll, for example, dolls wearing different clothes, if doll therapy is to be used by more than one person with dementia in the same unit. This will limit potential confusion over doll ownership – a doll should only belong to one person.

- Where possible and applicable, encourage family or care partners to bring in dolls that the person living with dementia may have previously owned.

- Avoid dolls that cry or that have their eyes closed. These have been shown to distress some people with dementia who engage with dolls, because they cannot stop their doll from crying or they believe their doll to be a baby that has died. There is currently no evidence to suggest one type of doll is more successful than another.

- Assist people with dementia to make their own choice about engaging with dolls; they should not be forced on everyone. Place the dolls in an area where people with dementia can make their own decisions (although this may be difficult if their mobility or sight is reduced).

- Keep accurate care plans relating to doll therapy. Monitoring levels of fatigue is particularly important, since caring for a doll as if it were a baby is tiring.

- If a person with dementia calls her doll by a certain name, all healthcare professionals and family members should be encouraged to do the same. And if the resident believes the doll to be a baby, this should not be invalidated.

- Never remove the doll without the permission of the person with dementia. When removing the doll, healthcare professionals and family members should hold the doll as if it was a living baby, and explain where they are taking the doll – for example, if it is dirty, the doll is going for a wash.

- Never remove the doll as a form of punishment. The person living with dementia may perceive the doll to be her child, and this can cause extreme distress.

- Do not place the doll in a box, on the floor or on a radiator, if storing the doll. It should be placed in a safe place, since the person engaging with the doll may perceive her 'baby' to be at risk.

Personalised care plan

Clara is an 80-year-old lady living with dementia. Clara currently enjoys engaging with doll therapy, and the following care plan has been informed by best practice evidence and was written up in consultation with Clara, her family and the extended healthcare team on the unit:

- At times Clara can experience episodes of distress.

- Clara is not currently prescribed any behaviour-modifying medication, as recommended by best practice evidence and global policy guidance.

- Pharmacological intervention may be necessary in the future if Clara's episodes of distress intensify over time, although this decision is considered a final resort.

- Presently Clara engages in numerous activities that are helpful at reducing episodes of distress and enhancing her overall wellbeing.

- One non-pharmacological approach that Clara particularly enjoys is doll therapy.

- Clara's family have been informed about Clara's enjoyment in using doll therapy, and are happy for this to be used as a therapeutic intervention. Clara's daughter and next of kin, Debbie, has signed a consent form for its use.

- Clara has named her doll 'Tom', and all care workers should refer to the doll as Tom because this validates Clara's experience.

- It is not clear whether Clara believes her doll, Tom, is a baby or a toy. Care staff should never refer to Tom as a doll or a baby. They should be guided by Clara and take her lead at all times. The important thing is to validate Clara's experiences.

- Clara engages with her doll, Tom, over a long period of time throughout the day. Care staff should ensure that Clara retains ownership of the doll at all times throughout the day, and not remove it without express consent from Clara.

- Clara likes to engage in a number of therapeutic activities with Tom, and these include washing, dressing, feeding, touching, stroking and cuddling the doll.

- Clara has not appeared distressed at any time when engaging with doll therapy, although all care staff must be mindful that this could change, and should continually monitor the therapeutic effect of doll therapy over time.

- If Clara is transferred to another unit, temporarily departs the unit or is admitted to another facility, then her doll, Tom, should accompany Clara at all times, because the separation may cause distress.

- This care plan should be evaluated a minimum of once per month with consideration of Clara's physical and emotional needs.

Educational framework

All care workers who help people living with dementia to derive therapeutic benefit from dolls should receive specialised education or training on their use. The following learning objectives should be covered so as to give care workers of all grades a comprehensive understanding of doll therapy in dementia care.

- Non-pharmacological approaches to dementia care:
  - understand the main types of non-pharmacological intervention in dementia care (e.g. music therapy, horticultural therapy, reminiscence therapy)
  - be aware that non-pharmacological approaches to dementia care should usually be tried before opting for pharmacological intervention
  - have knowledge about the importance of wellbeing, meaningful activity and person-centred care in dementia.

- The evidence base that underpins doll therapy:
  - understand that there is a growing empirical evidence base around the use of dolls in dementia care
  - have knowledge of the anecdotal evidence on doll therapy
  - know the variety of benefits that are associated with doll therapy (e.g. increased levels of communication, increased appetite and higher sustained wellbeing)
  - be aware of the challenges that are associated with delivery of doll therapy (e.g. stigma from people unfamiliar with the therapy and lack of education)
  - have knowledge on the main gaps in the doll therapy research.

- The theory behind doll therapy:
  - understand that there are a number of theories as to why doll therapy works, which may include Bowlby's theory of attachment or Winnicott's theory on transitional objects

- be aware that doll therapy is most commonly associated with fulfilment of attachment needs and results in profound paternal feelings.

- The ethics of doll therapy:

  - know that doll therapy is considered controversial in dementia care

  - be aware of the ethical principles and how these can be applied to doll therapy

  - have awareness of Kitwood's work on malignant social psychology and positive person work, as these may be applied to the practice of doll therapy.

- Best practice recommendations:

  - have an extensive knowledge of best practice recommendations in relation to the use of doll therapy in dementia care.

Conclusion

This chapter has provided a synopsis of best practice in relation to using doll therapy within a dementia care setting. The key components for introducing change in practice, and indeed change in attitude, relate to the introduction of a doll therapy policy, increasing awareness of the guidelines for using doll therapy in dementia care, encouraging healthcare professionals to develop personalised doll therapy care plans and administration of a structured education programme around the use of doll therapy in practice. By following these recommendations and including all the key components, it is more likely that doll therapy will not only be sustainable in the long term, but more successful for people living with dementia.

References

ADI (Alzheimer's Disease International) (2014) *World Alzheimer Report 2014: Dementia and Risk Reduction: An Analysis of Protective and Modifiable Factors.* London: ADI.

Alander, H., Prescott, T. and James, I. (2015) 'Older adults' views and experiences of doll therapy in residential care homes.' *Dementia 14*, 5, 574–588.

Andrew, A. (2006) 'The ethics of using dolls and soft toys in dementia care.' *Nursing and Residential Care 8*, 9, 419–421.

Baker, C. (2014) *Developing Excellent Care for People Living with Dementia in Care Homes.* London: Jessica Kingsley Publishers.

Ballard, C., Gauthier, S., Corbett, A., Brayne, C., Aarsland, D. and Jones, E. (2011) 'Alzheimer's disease', *The Lancet 377*, 9770, 1019–1031.

Banerjee, S. (2009) *The Use of Antipsychotic Medication for People with Dementia: Time for Action. A Report for the Minister of State for Care Services.* London: Department of Health.

Banerjee, S., Hellier, J., Romeo, R., Dewey, M. *et al.* (2013) 'Study of the use of antidepressants for depression in dementia: The HTA-SADD trial – a multicentre, randomised, double-blind, placebo-controlled trial of the clinical effectiveness and cost-effectiveness of sertraline and mirtazapine.' *Health Technology Assessment 17*, 7, 1–166.

Beauchamp, T. and Childress, J. (2009) *Principles of Biomedical Ethics* (6th edition). New York: Oxford University Press.

Bidewell, J. and Chang, E. (2014) 'Managing dementia agitation in residential aged care.' *Dementia 10*, 3, 299–315.

Bisiani, L. and Angus, J. (2013) 'Doll therapy: A therapeutic means to meet past attachment needs and diminish behaviours of concern in a person living with dementia – a case study approach.' *Dementia 12*, 4, 447–462.

Blake, M. and Mitchell, G. (2016) 'Horticultural therapy in dementia care: A literature review.' *Nursing Standard 30*, 21, 41–47.

Boas, I. (1998) 'Why do we have to give the name "therapy" to companionship and activities that are, or should be, a part of normal relationships?' *Journal of Dementia Care 6*, 6, 13.

Bowlby, J. (1969) *Attachment and Loss: Volume 1. Attachment.* London: Hogarth Press.

Braden, B. and Gaspar, P. (2015) 'Implementation of a baby doll therapy protocol for people with dementia (innovative practice).' *Dementia 14*, 5, 696–706.

Brooker, D. (2007) *Person-centred Dementia Care: Making Services Better*. London: Jessica Kingsley Publishers.

Butts, J. and Rich, K. (2008) *Nursing Ethics: Across the Curriculum and into Practice* (2nd edition). Sudbury, MA: Jones and Bartlett Publishers.

Chatterjee, J. (2012) 'Improving pain assessment for patients with cognitive impairment: Development of a pain assessment toolkit.' *International Journal of Palliative Nursing 18*, 12, 581–590.

Clarke, D. (2002) 'Between hope and acceptance: The medicalisation of dying.' *British Medical Journal 324*, 7342, 905–907.

Clarke, D. (2014) 'Palliative medicine as a specialty.' End of life studies. Available at http://endoflifestudies.academicblogs.co.uk/palliative-medicine-as-a-specialty, accessed on 27 February 2015.

Cohen-Mansfield, J. (2008) 'Use of patient characteristics to determine non-pharmacologic interventions for behavioural and psychological symptoms of dementia.' *International Psychogeriatrics 12*, suppl. 1, 373–380.

Cohen-Mansfield, J., Thein, K., Dakheel-Ali, M., Reiger, N. and Marx, S. (2010) 'The value of social attributes of stimuli for promoting engagement in persons with dementia.' *Journal of Nervous Mental Disorders 198*, 8, 586–592.

Culley, H., Barber, R., Hope, A. and James, I. (2013) 'Therapeutic lying in dementia care.' *Nursing Standard 28*, 1, 35–39.

Dewing, J. (2008) 'Personhood and dementia: Revisiting Tom Kitwood's ideas.' *International Journal of Older People Nursing 3*, 1, 3–13.

DH (Department of Health) (2008) *End of Life Care Strategy: Promoting High Quality of Care for All Adults at the End of Life*. London: DH.

DH (2009) *Living Well with Dementia: A National Dementia Strategy*. London: DH.

DH (2010) *Quality Outcomes for Patients with Dementia: Building on the Work of the National Dementia Strategy*. London: The Stationery Office.

DHSSPS (Department of Health, Social Services and Public Safety) (2010) *Living Matters, Dying Matters: The Northern Ireland Strategy for Palliative and End of Life Care*. Belfast: DHSSPS.

Division of Economic and Social Information and the Centre for Social Development and Humanitarian Affairs (1983) *World Programme of Action Concerning Disabled Persons*. New York: UN.

Draper, B. (2013) *Understanding Alzheimer's Disease and Other Dementias*. London: Jessica Kingsley Publishers.

Ellingford, J., Mackenzie, L. and Marsland, L. (2007) 'Using dolls to alter behaviour in patients with dementia.' *Nursing Times 103*, 5, 36–37.

Feil, N. (1982) *Validation: The Feil Method*. Cleveland, OH: Feil Productions.

Feil, N. (1993) *The Validation Breakthrough: Simple Techniques for Communicating with People with Alzheimer's-Type Dementia*. Baltimore, MD: Health Promotion Press.

Fraser, F. and James, I. (2008) 'Why does doll therapy improve the well-being of some older adults with dementia?' *PSIGE Newsletter 105*, October.

Freeman, M. (2011) *Human Rights: An Interdisciplinary Approach*. Cambridge: Polity Press.

Gold, K. (2014) 'But does it do any good? Measuring the impact of music therapy on people with advanced dementia (innovative practice).' *Dementia 13*, 2, 258–264.

Green, L., Matos, P., Murillo, I., Neushotz, L. *et al.* (2011) 'Use of dolls as a therapeutic intervention: Relationship to previous negative behaviors and pro re nata (PRN) Haldol use among geropsychiatric inpatients.' *Archives of Psychiatric Nursing 25*, 5, 388–389.

Harrison-Dening, K., Jones, L. and Sampson, E.L. (2011) 'Advance care planning for people with dementia: A review.' *International Psychogeriatrics 23*, 10, 1535–1551.

Heathcote, J. and Clare, M. (2014) 'Doll therapy: Therapeutic or childish or inappropriate?' *Nursing and Residential Care 16*, 1, 22–26.

Hughes, J., Jolley, D., Jordan, A. and Sampson, E. (2007) 'Palliative care in dementia: Issues and evidence.' *Advances in Psychiatric Treatment 13*, 251–260.

James, I. (2011) *Understanding Behaviour in Dementia that Challenges: A Guide to Assessment and* Treatment. London: Jessica Kingsley Publishers.

James, I., Mackenzie, L. and Mukaetova-Ladinska, E. (2006) 'Doll use in care homes for people with dementia.' *International Journal of Geriatric Psychiatry 21*, 1093–1098.

James, I., Mackenzie, L., Pakrasi, S. and Fossey, J. (2008) 'Non-pharmacological treatments of challenging behaviour.' *Nursing and Residential Care 10*, 5, 228–232.

Johnstone, M. (2006) *Bioethics: A Nursing Perspective* (4th edition). London: Churchill Livingstone.

Jones, S. and Mitchell, G. (2015) 'Assessment of pain and alleviation of distress for people living with a dementia.' *Mental Health Practice 18*, 10, 32–36.

Kelly, F. and Innes, A. (2013) 'Human rights, citizenship and dementia care nursing.' *International Journal of Older People Nursing 8*, 1, 61–70.

Kitwood, T. (1993) 'Towards a theory of dementia care: The interpersonal process.' *Ageing and Society 13*, 51–67.

Kitwood, T. (1995) 'Positive long-term changes in dementia: Some preliminary observations.' *Journal of Mental Health 4*, 133–144.

Kitwood, T. (1997) *Dementia Reconsidered: The Person Comes First*. Buckingham: Open University Press.

Loboprabhu, S., Molinari, V. and Lomax, J. (2007) 'The transitional object in dementia: Clinical implications.' *International Journal of Applied Psychoanalytic Studies 4*, 144–169.

Locke, J. (1997) *An Essay Concerning Human Understanding*. Harmondsworth: Penguin Books.

Lunney, J., Lynn, J., Foley, D., Lipson, S. and Guralnik, J. (2003) 'Patterns of functional decline at the end of life.' *JAMA: Journal of the American Medical Assocation 289*, 18, 2387–2392.

Mackenzie, L., Wood-Mitchell, A. and James, I (2007) 'Guidelines on using dolls.' *Journal of Dementia Care 15*, 1, 26–27.

Mackenzie, L., James, I., Morse, R., Mukaetova-Ladinska, E. and Reichelt, K. (2006) 'A pilot study on the use of dolls for people with dementia.' *Age and Ageing 35*, 4, 441–444.

McCormack, B. (2003) 'A conceptual framework for person-centred practice with older people.' *International Journal of Nursing Practice 9*, 202–209.

McCormack, B. and McCance, T. (2006) 'Development of a framework for person-centred nursing.' *Journal of Advanced Nursing 56*, 1–18.

McCormack, B. and McCance, T. (2010) *Person-centred Nursing: Theory and Practice.* Oxford: Wiley Blackwell.

McCormack, B., Dewing, J. and McCance, T. (2011) 'Developing person-centred care: Addressing contextual challenges through practice development.' *OJIN: Online Journal of Issues in Nursing 16*, 2, Manuscript 3.

McCormack, B., Karlsson, B., Dewing, J. and Lerdal, A. (2010a) 'Exploring personcentredness: A qualitative meta-synthesis of four studies.' *Scandinavian Journal of Caring Sciences 24*, 620–634.

McCormack, B., Dewing, J., Breslin, L., Coyne-Nevin, A., Kennedy, K., Manning, M. and Slater, P. (2010b) 'Developing person-centred practice: Nursing outcomes arising from changes to the care environment in residential settings for older people.' *International Journal of Older People Nursing 5*, 93–107.

McCormack, B., Roberts, T., Meyer, J., Morgan, D. and Boscart, V. (2012) 'Appreciating the person in long-term care.' *International Journal of Older People Nursing 7*, 284–294.

McGreevy, J. (2016) 'Implementing culture change in long-term dementia care settings.' *Nursing Standard 30*, 19, 44–50.

McIlfatrick, S., Noble, H., McCorry, N.K., Roulston, A. *et al.* (2014) 'Exploring public awareness and perceptions of palliative care: A qualitative study.' *Palliative Medicine 28*, 3, 273–280.

McNamara, B., Rosenwax, L.K. and Holman, C.D.J. (2006) 'A method for defining and estimating the palliative care population.' *Journal of Pain and Symptom Management 32*, 1, 5–12.

Miesen, B. (1993) 'Alzheimer's disease, the phenomenon of parent fixation and Bowlby's attachment theory.' *International Journal of Geriatric Psychiatry 8*, 147–153.

Minshull, K. (2009) 'The impact of doll therapy on well-being of people with dementia.' *Journal of Dementia Care 17*, 2, 35–38.

Mitchell, G. (2013) 'Applying pharmacology to practice: The case of dementia.' *Nurse Prescribing 11*, 4, 185–190.

Mitchell, G. (2014a) 'Use of doll therapy for people with dementia: An overview.' *Nursing Older People 26*, 4, 24–26.

Mitchell, G. (2014b) 'Therapeutic lying to assist people with dementia in maintaining medication adherence.' *Nursing Ethics 21*, 7, 844–845.

Mitchell, G. (2015) 'Palliative and end-of-life decision-making in dementia care.' *International Journal of Palliative Nursing 21*, 11, 536–541.

Mitchell, G. and Agnelli, J. (2015a) 'Non-pharmacological approaches to alleviate distress in dementia care.' *Nursing Standard 30*, 13, 38–44.

Mitchell, G. and Agnelli, J. (2015b) 'Person-centred care for people with dementia: Kitwood reconsidered.' *Nursing Standard 30*, 7, 46–50.

Mitchell, G. and O'Donnell, H. (2013) 'The therapeutic use of doll therapy in dementia.' *British Journal of Nursing 22*, 6, 329–334.

Mitchell, G. and Templeton, M. (2014) 'Ethical considerations of doll therapy for people with dementia.' *Nursing Ethics 21*, 6, 720–730.

Mitchell, G. and Twycross, A. (2015) 'Optimising palliative and end of life care in care home settings.' *Evidence Based Nursing 19*, 1, 1.

Mitchell, G., McCollum, P. and Monaghan, C. (2013a) 'The personal impact of disclosure of a dementia diagnosis: A thematic review of the literature.' *British Journal of Neuroscience Nursing 9*, 5, 223–228.

Mitchell, G., McCollum, P. and Monaghan, C. (2013b) 'Disclosing a diagnosis of dementia: A background to the phenomenon.' *Nursing Older People 25*, 10, 16–21.

Mitchell, G., McCormack, B. and McCance, T. (2014) 'Therapeutic use of dolls for people living with dementia: A critical review of the literature.' *Dementia*, 1–26. doi: 10.1177/1471301214548522

Mitchell, G., Agnelli, J., McGreevy, J., Diamond, M., Roble, H., McShane, E. and Strain, J. (2016) 'Optimum delivery of palliative and end of life care for people living with dementia in care home settings.' *Nursing Standard* (in press).

Moore, D. (2001) 'It's like a gold medal and it's mine – dolls in dementia care.' *Journal of Dementia Care 9*, 6, 20–23.

Moniz-Cook, E. (2006) 'Cognitive stimulation and dementia.' *Ageing and Mental Health 10*, 3, 207–210.

Murtagh, F.E.M., Preston, M. and Higginson, I. (2004) 'Patterns of dying: Palliative care for non-malignant disease.' *Professional Issues 4*, 1, 39–44.

NCPC (National Council for Palliative Care) (2006) *Introductory Guide to End of Life Care in Care Homes*. Leicester: NCPC and NHS End of Life Care Programme.

NCPC (2009) *End of Life Care Manifesto 2010*. London: NCPC.

NHPCO (National Hospice and Palliative Care Organization) (2013) *NHPCO's Facts and Figures: Hospice Care in America*. Alexandria, VA: NHPCO.

NICE (National Institute for Health and Clinical Excellence) (2006) *Dementia: Supporting People with Dementia and their Carers in Health and Social Care*. Clinical Guideline 42. London: NICE.

NICE (2011) *Quality Standard for End of Life Care for Adults*. London: NICE.

NICE (2011) *A NICE–SCIE Guideline on Supporting People with Dementia and Their Carers in Health and Social Care*. National Clinical Practice Guideline Number 42. London: HMSO.

Nolan, M., Brown, J., Davies, S., Nolan, J. and Keady, J. (2006) *The Senses Framework: Improving Care for Older People through a Relationship-centred Approach*. Getting Research into Practice (GRiP) Report No. 2. Sheffield: University of Sheffield.

Perez-Merino, R. (2014) 'Strategies for enhancing the delivery of person-centred care.' *Nursing Standard 28*, 39, 37–41.

Pezzati, R., Molteni, V., Bani, M., Settanta, C. *et al.* (2014) 'Can doll therapy preserve or promote attachment in people with cognitive, behavioural, and emotional problems? A pilot study in institutionalized patients with dementia.' *Frontiers in Psychology 5*, 342, 1–9.

Rahman, S. (2014) *Living Well with Dementia: The Importance of the Person and the Environment for Wellbeing.* New York: Radcliffe Publishing.

Roger, K. (2006) 'A literature review of palliative care, end of life and dementia.' *Palliative and Supportive Care 4*, 295–303.

Rogers, C. (1961) *On Becoming a Person.* Boston, MA: Houghton Mifflin.

Roper, N., Logan, W. and Tierney, A. (2000) *The Roper-Logan-Tierney Model for Nursing: Based on the Activities of Living.* Edinburgh: Churchill Livingstone.

Salari, S. (2002) 'Intergenerational partnerships in adult day centres: Importance of age-appropriate environments and behaviours.' *The Gerontologist 42*, 321–333.

Schermer, M. (2007) 'Nothing but the truth? On truth and deception in dementia care.' *Bioethics 21*, 1, 13–22.

Sepulveda, C., Marlin, A., Yoshida, T. and Ullrich, A. (2002) 'Palliative care: The World Health Organization's global perspective.' *Journal of Pain and Symptom Management 24*, 2, 91–96.

Shin, J. (2015) 'Doll therapy: An intervention for nursing home residents with dementia.' *Journal of Psychosocial Nursing and Mental Health Services 53*, 1, 13–18.

Steenbergen, E., Smith, C., Bright, C. and Kaaijik, M. (2013) 'Perspectives of person-centred care.' *Nursing Standard 27*, 48, 35–41.

Stephens, A., Cheston, R. and Gleeson, K. (2013) 'An exploration into the relationships people with dementia have with physical objects: An ethnographic study.' *Dementia 12*, 6, 697–712.

Sturdy, D., Heath, H., Ballard, C. and Burns, A. (2012) *Antipsychotic Drugs in Dementia: A Best Practice Guide.* Harrow on the Hill: RCN Publishing Company.

Swaffer, K. (2014) 'Dementia: Stigma, language, and dementia-friendly.' *Dementia 13*, 6, 709–716.

Tamura, T., Nakajima, K. and Nambu., M. (2001) 'Baby dolls as therapeutic tools for severe dementia patients.' *International Journal of Gerontechnology 1*, 2, 111–118.

Tuckett, A. (1998) 'Code of ethics: Assistance with a lie choice?' *Australian Journal of Holistic Nursing 5*, 2, 36–40.

Tuckett, A. (2012) 'The experience of lying in dementia care: A qualitative study.' *Nursing Ethics 19*, 1, 7–20.

UN General Assembly (2007) *Convention on the Rights of Persons with Disabilities.* Resolution adopted by the General Assembly, 24 January, A/RES/61/106. Available at www.refworld.org/docid/45f973632.html, accessed on 1 September 2015.

van der Steen, J.T., Radbruch, L., Hertogh, C.M.P.H., de Boer, M.E. *et al.* (2014) 'White paper defining optimal palliative care in older people with dementia: A Delphi study and recommendations from the European Association for Palliative Care.' *Palliative Medicine 28*, 3, 197–209.

Verity, J. (2006) 'Dolls in dementia care: Bridging the divide.' *Journal of Dementia Care 14*, 1, 25–27.

Winnicott, W. (1953) 'Traditional objects and transitional phenomena: A study of the first not-me possession.' *The International Journal of Psychoanalysis 34*, 89–97.

Wood-Mitchell, A., James, I., Waterworth, A., Swann, A. and Ballard, C. (2008) 'Factors influencing the prescribing of medications by old age physiatrists for behavioural and psychological symptoms of dementia: A qualitative study.' *Age and Ageing 37*, 5, 547–552.

Woods, B., Aguirre, E, Spector, A. and Orrell, M. (2012) 'Cognitive stimulation to improve cognitive functioning in people with dementia.' *Cochrane Database of Systematic Reviews 2*, Art No. CD005562.

WHO (World Health Organization) (1996) *Cancer Pain Relief. With a Guide to Opioid Availability* (2nd edition). Geneva, Switzerland: WHO.

WHO (2002) *WHO Definition of Palliative Care*. Available at www.who.int/cancer/palliative/definition/en, accessed on 25 February 2015.

WHO (2004) *Palliative Care: The Solid Facts*. Copenhagen, Denmark: WHO.

WHO (2007) *Cancer Control: Knowledge into Action. WHO Guide for Effective Programmes*. Geneva, Switzerland: WHO.

WHO (2014) *Global Atlas of Palliative Care at the End of Life*. London: WHO and Worldwide Palliative Care Alliance.

Wynne, L. (2013) 'Spiritual care at end of life.' *Nursing Standard 28*, 2, 41–45.

Index

Page references to Figures or Tables are in *italics*

CPSIA information can be obtained
at www.ICGtesting.com
Printed in the USA
FFOW05n1743110716

9 781849 055703